Second MBBS Buster
PHARMACOLOGY

Second MBBS Buster
PHARMACOLOGY

Editors

Avishek Layek MBBS (Gold Medalist)
Internee, Nil Ratan Sircar Medical College and Hospital
Kolkata, West Bengal, India

Dyuti Deepta Rano MBBS (Gold Medalist)
Internee, Nil Ratan Sircar Medical College and Hospital
Kolkata, West Bengal, India

Foreword
Nilanjan Sengupta

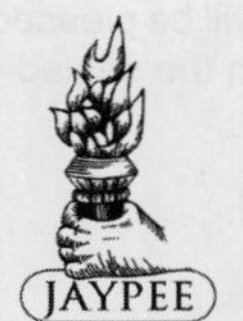

JAYPEE The Health Sciences Publisher

New Delhi | London | Panama

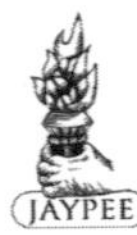

Jaypee Brothers Medical Publishers (P) Ltd.

Headquarters
Jaypee Brothers Medical Publishers (P) Ltd.
4838/24, Ansari Road, Daryaganj
New Delhi 110 002, India
Phone: +91-11-43574357
Fax: +91-11-43574314
E-mail: jaypee@jaypeebrothers.com

Overseas Offices
J.P. Medical Ltd.
83, Victoria Street, London
SW1H 0HW (UK)
Phone: +44-20 3170 8910
Fax: +44(0)20 3008 6180
E-mail: info@jpmedpub.com

Jaypee-Highlights Medical Publishers Inc.
City of Knowledge, Bld. 235, 2nd Floor, Clayton
Panama City, Panama
Phone: +1 507-301-0496
Fax: +1 507-301-0499
E-mail: cservice@jphmedical.com

Jaypee Brothers Medical Publishers (P) Ltd.
17/1-B, Babar Road, Block-B, Shyamoli
Mohammadpur, Dhaka-1207
Bangladesh
Mobile: +08801912003485
E-mail: jaypeedhaka@gmail.com

Jaypee Brothers Medical Publishers (P) Ltd.
Bhotahity, Kathmandu, Nepal
Phone: +977-9741283608
E-mail: kathmandu@jaypeebrothers.com

Website: www.jaypeebrothers.com
Website: www.jaypeedigital.com

Inquiries for bulk sales may be solicited at: jaypee@jaypeebrothers.com

Second MBBS Buster Pharmacology

First Edition: **2018**

ISBN: 978-93-5270-489-7

Printed at Rajkamal Electric Press, Plot No. 2, Phase-IV, Kundli, Haryana.

Dedicated to

Our Parents

&

All Second Professional MBBS Students!

Contributors

Anusree Krishna Mandal MBBS (Honors)
Internee, Nil Ratan Sircar Medical College and Hospital
Kolkata, West Bengal, India

Arnab Pal
Internee, Nil Ratan Sircar Medical College and Hospital
Kolkata, West Bengal, India

Avishek Layek MBBS (Gold Medalist)
Internee, Nil Ratan Sircar Medical College and Hospital
Kolkata, West Bengal, India

Dyuti Deepta Rano MBBS (Gold Medalist)
Internee, Nil Ratan Sircar Medical College and Hospital
Kolkata, West Bengal, India

Tathagata Bhattacharya
Internee, Nil Ratan Sircar Medical College and Hospital
Kolkata, West Bengal, India

Foreword

Second MBBS Buster Pharmacology is a unique handbook for the undergraduate students preparing for Pharmacology examination of West Bengal University of Health Sciences (and, for that matter, other universities too). Needless to mention, this is never a substitute to full-fledged textbook of pharmacology but an invaluable supplement to the same. The handbook is unique because it is compiled by two young medicos who appeared successfully in the Pharmacology examination not too long back. Hence, the book is designed primarily keeping in mind the deficits of a standard textbook, the lacunae in conventional teaching, and the practical problems a beginner faces.

The chapters, better to be described as sections, though not comprehensive, are practically oriented helping the students prepare for topics like long questions, short notes, prescription writing, prescription criticism, drug interactions and chart interpretations to help sail through the practical examination. Additionally a chapter is dedicated to guide through the oral examination.

Thus, the authors have attempted to present to the students of pharmacology a 360 degree view of the present examination format and what are expected of them in the examination.

This handbook, a first of its kind in this part of the country, should be a very useful companion to students and will aid in a scientific and practical approach towards preparation for the examination. A must read for all Second MBBS students.

Nilanjan Sengupta
Professor and Head
Department of Endocrinology
Nil Ratan Sircar Medical College and Hospital
Kolkata, West Bengal, India

Preface

At the outset we humbly beg to state that this book is not a textbook of pharmacology, but merely an aid that would make preparation of pharmacology Second Professional MBBS examination easier. When we started of reading Pharmacology in our 3rd semester, in the winter of 2014; it was barely three weeks for our internal assessment examinations. While preparing for the same we felt the dire need of a student friendly and oriented book that could smoothen the examination preparation process. We started analyzing and decoding question paper patterns and writing answers; the compilation of our 3rd, 4th and 5th semester notes, which we now humbly present to you as our first published book. Our ambition has always been to be an author from a student's perspective. We have included the viva voce questions from the experiences of our own and our acquaintances. The values have been adopted from standard references and format has been kept such that is easily reproducible in examinations. Hence, this book shall not only be some inked pages with a cover, but a friend in need—and a true one indeed.

Avishek Layek

Dyuti Deepta Rano

Acknowledgments

First of all, we would like to thank our parents and dear ones for all their support and love. Their blessings and support have made this possible.

We would like to thank our faculties from the Department of Pharmacology, Nil Ratan Sircar Medical College and Hospital, Kolkata, West Bengal, India for all their good wishes and help throughout writing the book; especially Professor Drs Nina Das, Tania Sur Kundu, Parama Sengupta, Subir Mukhopadhyay and Tanmoy Goswami.

We are extremely grateful to our juniors Satyaki and Chayan, Seniors Dr SM Isha and Nur Nabab Mollah for the constant support during our maiden voyage.

We shall be indebted to the authors of the following books that helped us in crafting the model answers: *Essentials of Medical Pharmacology (KD Tripathi), Goodman and Gilman's The Pharmacological Basis of Therapeutics, Pharmacology for Second Professional Students (MM Das) and Harrison's Principles of Internal Medicine.*

We would like to thank Deblina Chatterjee who was the first person to incept us with the idea of converting our notes into a book that could possibly benefit batches to come.

We thank all our friends and juniors who read our answers and suggested their valuable edits specially Nivedita and Arkaprabha.

Last but not least, we extend our humble regards and gratitude to all students and teachers of our profession.

Contents

Pattern of Pharmacology Examination in 2nd Professional MBBS

Total 150 marks

PHARMACOLOGY THEORY: 2 PAPERS OF 40 MARKS EACH = TOTAL 80

PATTERN OF THEORY PAPER

Group A: Long question. 10 marks (one out of two)
Group B: Explain why. 3 × 3=9 (three out of four)
Group C: Mechanism of action. 3 × 3= 9 (three out of four)
Group D: Short notes. 3 × 4 = 12 (four out of five)

PHARMACOLOGY GRAND VIVA: Total 15 marks

PHARMACOLOGY INTERNAL ASSESSMENT:
Theory 15 Marks + Practical 15 Marks = Total 30

PHARMACOLOGY PRACTICAL: Total 25 marks

	Total
1. Prescription-one	
Format	1
Writing	1
Oral crossing	2
Total:	**4**
2. Pharmacy- one item	
Preparation and labeling	2
Oral crossing	2
Total:	**4**
3. Therapeutic Problem-one	
Correct interpretation of therapeutic situation in writing	2
Oral crossing	2
Total:	**4**
4. Drug Interaction-one	
Interpretation in writing	2
Oral crossing	2
Total:	**4**

5. Experimental Pharmacology	
Charts/graphs and diagrams	Interpretation-2 Interpretation-2
Total:	**4**
6. Sample-based-knowledge testing (spotting)	**2**
7. Criticism of prescription	**3** (Oral table)
Total	**25**

Practical Notebooks—Two

One: Therapeutics Record Book—Containing patterns utilization of drugs in emergency and inpatient departments.
One: Pharmacy.

Practical notebooks must be submitted in practical examination—without which students are **NOT ALLOWED** to appear.

CHAPTER

1

Definitions in Pharmacology

Avishek Layek

- **Drug**: Drug is any substance or product that is used or is intended to be used to modify or explore physiological systems or pathological states for the benefit of the recipient.
  Drugs thus can be classified according to this definition into four basic types:
  i. Modify physiological system, e.g. vaccines modifying immune system
  ii. Explore physiological system, e.g. radioiodine dyes to exclude pathology
  iii. Modify pathological system, e.g. diuretic to reverse edema
  iv. Explore pathological system, e.g. radioactive dyes to confirm pathology.
- **Pharmacokinetics**: It is defined as movement of the drug in and alteration of the drug by the body; including absorption, binding/localization/storage, biotransformation and excretion of the drug.
- **Pharmacodynamics**: It is defined as the study of the biochemical and physiological effects of drugs and their mechanisms of action at organ system/subcellular/macromolecular levels.
- **Chemotherapy**: It is defined as the treatment of systemic infections or malignancy with specific drugs that have selective toxicity for the infecting organism or malignant cell respectively, with no or minimal effects on the host cell.
  Another classification of drugs may be:
  - Pharmacodynamics agents—designed to have pharmacodynamics effects in the recipient
  - Chemotherapeutic agents—inhibit or kill parasite/malignant cell with minimal pharmacodynamics effect to the recipient (however, there is no drug that has zero systemic effect).
- **Essential medicines**: They are defined as those drugs that satisfy the priority healthcare needs of the population. They are selected with due regard to public health relevance, evidence on efficacy and safety and comparative cost effectiveness.
  No. of essential drugs in National List of Essential Medicines of India:
  - 2011 : 348
  - 2015 : 376 (106 drugs added and 70 deleted from 2011 list)
- **Orphan drugs**: These are drugs or biological products for diagnosis or treatment or prevention of a rare disease or condition, or a more common disease (endemic only in resource poor countries) for which there is reasonable expectation that the cost of developing and marketing it will be recovered from the sales of that drug, e.g.:
  - Sodium nitrite—used with sodium thiosulfate to treat cyanide poisoning
  - Fomepizole—treat methanol and ethylene glycol poisoning
  - Liposomal amphotericin B—used in morbid systemic fungal infections

- **Bioavailability**: Defined as the rate and extent of absorption of a drug from a dosage form which is measure of the fraction of administered dose of the drug that reaches the systemic circulation in unchanged form.
  - 100% bioavailability is attained in intravenous route.
    Exception: Chloramphenicol succinate; about 70% because renal excretion of ester before hydrolysis.
  - Nearly 100% oral bioavailability is attained in levofloxacin.

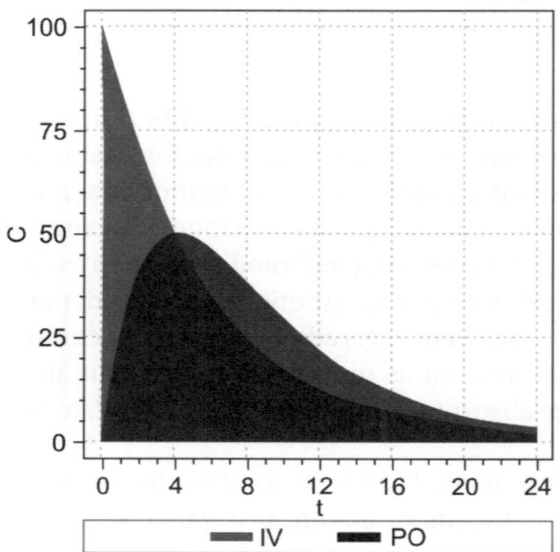

Fig. 1.1: Concentration-time graph showing bioavailability for IV and oral routes

- **Apparent volume of distribution**: Presuming that the body behaves as a single homogeneous compartment, the apparent volume of distribution is defined as the volume that would accommodate all the drug in the body; if the concentration throughout was the same as plasma.

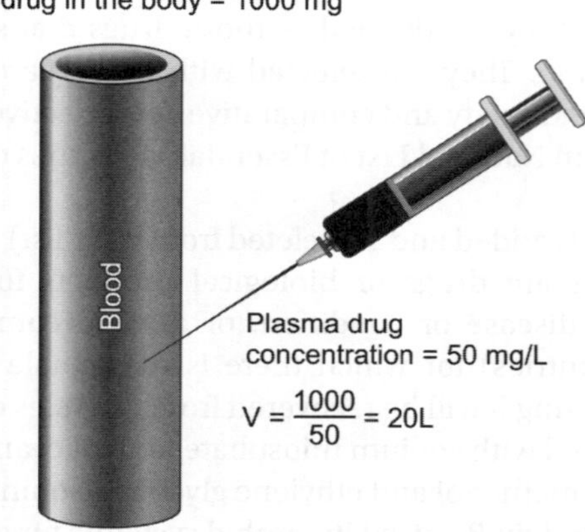

Fig. 1.2: The concept of apparent volume of distribution in one compartment model

- **Biotransformation**: Defined as the chemical alteration of blood in the body. Isoniazid undergoes phase II followed by phase I reaction.
- **Clearance:** It is defined as the theoretical volume of plasma from which the drug is completely removed in unit time.
    - Phenytoin/tolbutamide/theophylline/warfarin initially show zero order but then follow 1st order kinetics
    - Ethyl alcohol follows zero order kinetics.

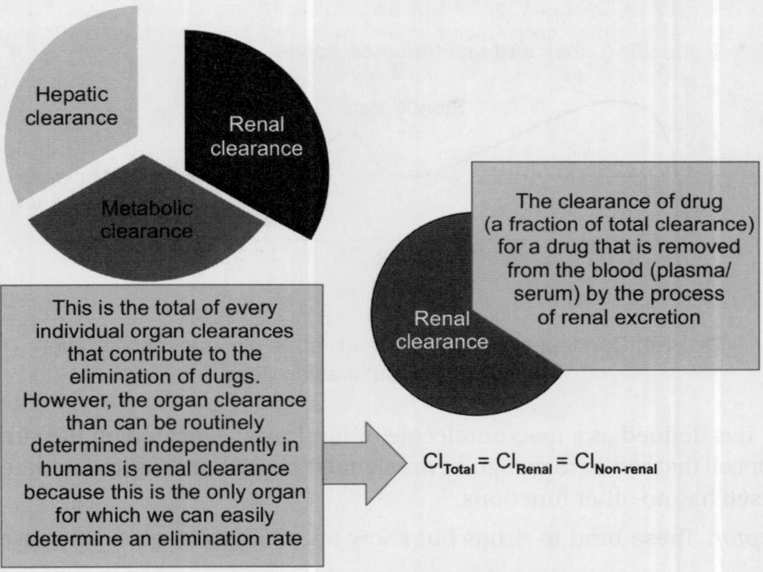

Fig. 1.3: The concept of clearance of a drug's

- **Half-life**:
    - *Plasma half-life*: It is the time taken for the plasma concentration of the drug to be reduced to half from its original value
    - *Biological effect of peak effect half-life*: The time in which pharmacological effect of a drug or its active metabolites is reduced to half
    - *Elimination half-life*: The time in which the total amount of the drug in the body after equilibrium is attained (in plasma, fat, muscle, etc.) is reduced to half
    - *Hit and run drugs*: Drugs whose peak effect half-life > elimination half-life, e.g. proton pump inhibitors, monoamine oxidase inhibitors.
- **Loading dose**: This is a single or few quickly repeated doses given in the beginning to attain target concentration rapidly.
- **Maintenance dose**: This dose is one that is to be repeated at specific intervals after the attainment of target steady state plasma concentration so as to maintain the same by balancing elimination.

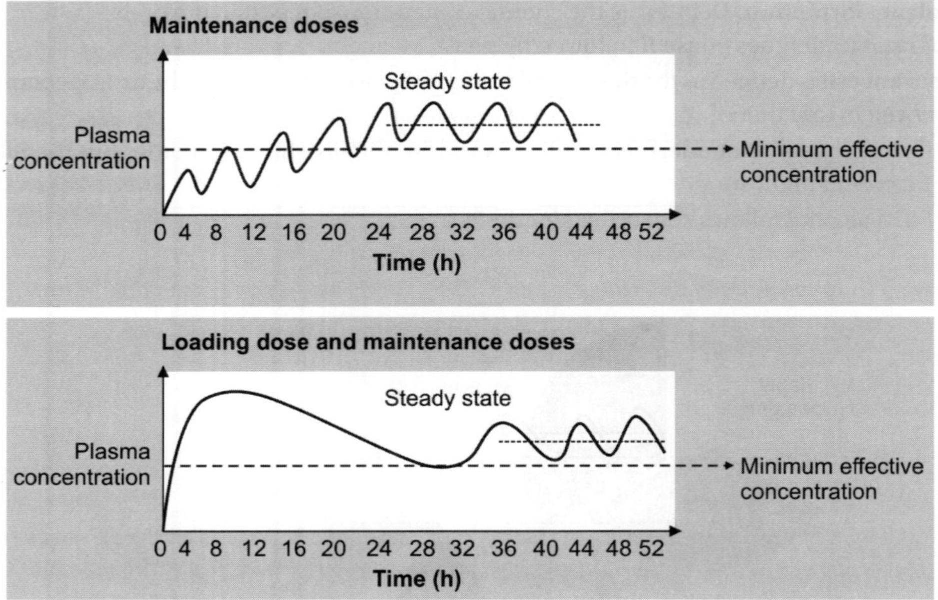

Fig. 1.4: Concept of achieving steady state plasma concentration with and without loading dose

- **Receptor**: It is defined as a macromolecule or binding site located on the surface or inside the effector cell that serves to recognize the signal molecule or drug and initiate the response to it, but itself has no other functions.

  Silent receptor: These bind to drugs but show no pharmacological response, e.g. plasma proteins.
- **Agonist**: An agent which activates a receptor to produce an effect similar to that of the physiological signal molecule. (Affinity is present and intrinsic activity = +1) (e.g. adrenaline at alpha adrenergic receptor, histamine at H1 receptor, etc.).
- **Antagonist**: An agent which prevents the action of an agonist on a receptor or the subsequent response, but does not have any effect of its own (affinity is present and intrinsic activity = 0) (propranolol at beta-adrenergic receptors).
- **Inverse agonist**: An agent which activates a receptor to produce an effect in the opposite direction to that of the agonist (affinity present and intrinsic activity = –1 to 0) (DMCM on BZD receptor).
- **Partial agonist**: An agent which activates a receptor to produce submaximal effect, but antagonizes the action of a full agonist (affinity present and intrinsic activity = 0 to +1) (Dichloroisoproterenol on beta-adrenergic receptors).
- **Ligand**: Any molecule which attaches selectively to particular receptors or sites.
- **Antagonism**:
  - *Competitive or equilibrium type*: Increased kM but V_{max} is unchanged, e.g. Methotrexate on dihydrofolate reductase
  - *Noncompetitive type*: kM remains unchanged but V_{max} is reduced, e.g. aspirin on COX.

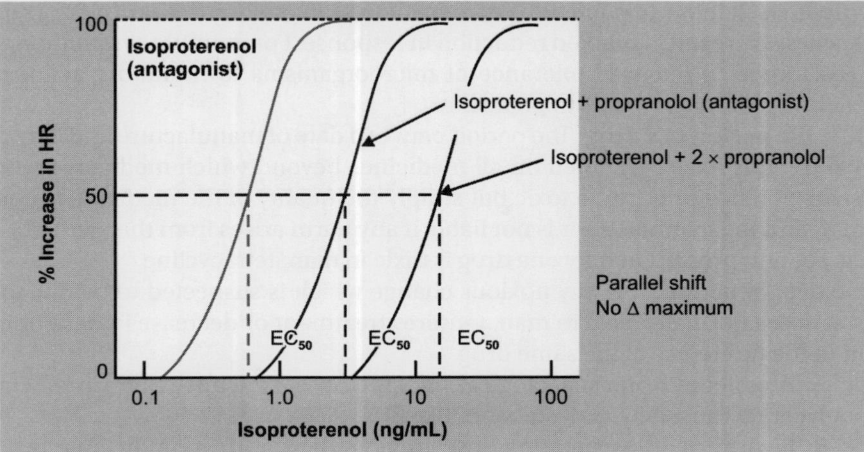

Fig. 1.5: Competitive antagonism

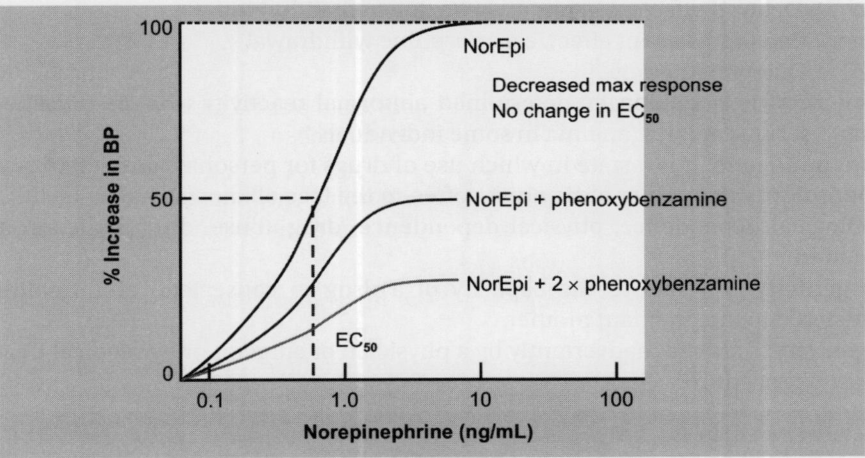

Fig. 1.6: Noncompetitive antagonism

- **Fixed dose combination**: A single formulation containing 2 or more drugs in a fixed dose ratio. NLEM India 2011 approves only 12 FDCs where as WHO approves 23 of them. Most widely used FDC is ORS.
- **Placebo**: This is an inert substance given in the garb of medicine which works by psychodynamics rather than pharmacodynamics means.
  Naloxone suppresses endorphins in brain and can antagonize psychodynamics effect too.
- **Tolerance**: It refers to the requirement of higher doses of a drug to produce a given response, e. g. sulfonylureas in type 2 DM.
- **Cross tolerance**: It is a development of tolerance to pharmacologically related drugs, e. g. alcoholics are relatively resistant to barbiturates and general anesthetics.
- **Intolerance**: It is the appearance of characteristic toxic effects of a drug in an individual at therapeutic doses. For example, carbamazepine producing ataxia in some people.

- **Tachyphylaxis**: It refers to rapid development of tolerance when doses of a drug repeated in quick succession result in marked reduction in response. For example, tyramine, ephedrine.
- **Drug resistance**: It refers to tolerance of microorganisms to inhibitory actions of antimicrobials, e.g. *Staphylococcus* to penicillin.
- **Shelf life/life period of a drug**: The period between date of manufacture and date of expiry.
- **Expiry date**: It is a date stamped on all medicines beyond which medicine actually does not lose its potency or become toxic but simply the quality of the medicine is not assured beyond it; and the manufacturer is not liable if any harm arises from the use of it.
  The degradation product of only one drug is toxic in man: tetracycline
- **Adverse drug reaction**: It is any noxious change which is suspected to be due to a drug , occurs at doses normally used in man, requires treatment or decrease in dose or indicated caution in the future use of the same drug.
  - *Type A:* Augmented pharmacological effects—dose dependent and predictable, e.g. hypoglycemia caused by anti-diabetics like SUs.
  - *Type B:* Bizarre or idiosyncratic—dose independent and unpredictable, e.g. allergic reaction to penicillins
  - *Type C:* Chronic effects, e.g. peptic ulcer due to NSAIDs
  - *Type D:* Delayed effects, e.g. phocomelia due to thalidomide
  - *Type E:* End of treatment effect, e.g. morphine withdrawal
  - *Type F:* Failure of therapy.
- **Idiosyncrasy**: It is genetically determined abnormal reactivity to a chemical, e. g. dose unrelated serious aplastic anemia in some individuals.
- **Drug dependence**: It is a state in which use of drugs for personal satisfaction is accorded a higher priority than other basic needs, often in the face of known risks to health. Types—psychological dependence, physical dependence, drug abuse, drug addiction and drug habituation.
- **Teratogenicity**: It refers to the capacity of a drug to cause fetal abnormalities when administered to the pregnant mother.
- **Iatrogenicity**: Induced inadvertently by a physician or surgeon or by medical treatment or diagnostic procedures.

Risk category of drugs during pregnancy		
Category		*Examples*
A	Adequate studies in pregnant women have failed to demonstrate a risk to the fetus	Inj. Mag. sulfate, thyroxine
B	Adequate human studies are lacking, but animal studies have failed to demonstrate a risk to the fetus or Adequate studies in pregnant women have failed to demonstrate a risk to the fetus, but animal studies have shown an adverse effect on the fetus	Penicillin V, amoxicillin, cefaclor, erythromycin, paracetamol, lignocaine
C	No adequate studies in pregnant women and animal studies are lacking or have shown and adverse effect on fetus, but potential benefit may warrant use of the drug in pregnant women despite potential risk	Morphine, codeine, atropine, corticosteroids, adrenaline, thiopentone, bupivacaine
D	There is evidence of human fetal risk, but the potential benefits from use of the drug may be acceptable despite the potential risk	Aspirin, phenytoin, carbamazepine, valproate, lorazepam
X	Studies in animals or humans have demonstrated fetal abnormalities, and potential risk clearly outweigh possible benefit	Estrogens, isotretinoin, ergometrine

- **Pharmacovigilance**: Defined by WHO in 2002 as the science and activities relating to the detection, assessment, understanding and prevention of adverse effects or any other drug related problems.
- **Therapeutic window phenomenon**: Some drugs show sub-optimal efficacy below a certain concentration and also beyond a certain concentration. Classical example is clonidine which shows optimum BP lowering between blood levels of 0.2 to 2.0 ng/mL.
- **Clinical trial**: According to WHO, clinical trial is any research study that prospectively assigns human participants or groups of humans to one or more health related interventions to evaluate the effects on health outcomes. Summary of clinical trials:

Phase	*Name*	*Conducted on*	*Blinding and control*	*Purpose*
I	Human pharmacology and safety	Healthy volunteers (20–100)	Open Label (No binding)	• To know maximum tolerable dose (MTD) • Safety and tolerability
II	Therapeutic exploratory	100–150 patients (homogeneous population)	Single blind controlled	• To establish therapeutic efficacy • Dose ranging and ceiling effect
III	Therapeutic confirmatory	Up to 5000 patients from several centers (heterogeneous population)	Double blind randomized controlled	• To confirm therapeutic efficacy • To establish the value of drug in relation to existing therapy
IV	Post-marketing surveillance	Large number of patients being treated by practicing physicians	—	• To know rare and long-term adverse effects • Special groups like children, pregnancy, etc. can be tested
0 (Zero)	Microdosing studies	Healthy volunteers (small number)	–	Very low dose 1/100 of human dose; max 100 mg of drug is administered to know pharmacokinetics. This could avoid costly phase I studies for candidate drugs with unsuitable pharmacokinetics

- **Autacoids**: These are diverse substances produced by a wide variety of cells in the body, having intense biological activities but generally act locally (e.g. within inflammatory pockets) at the site of synthesis and release. The classical autacoids are: amine autacoids (histamine, 5-HT), lipid derived autacoids (PGs, leukotrienes, PAFs) and peptide autacoids (bradykinin, angiotensin).
- **Bronchial asthma**: It is a heterogeneous disease, usually characterized by chronic airway inflammation. It is defined by the history of respiratory symptoms such as wheeze, shortness of breath, chest tightness and cough that vary over time and in intensity, together with variable expiratory airflow limitation (GINA).
- **Status asthmaticus**: It is a life threatening acute exacerbation of bronchial asthma wherein bronchospasm is not relieved with aggressive therapy within 30–60 minutes and attacks follow without any pause.

  Blood gas progression in status asthmaticus:
  - *Stage 1*: Hyperventilation (low PCO_2) with a normal (PO_2).

- *Stage 2*: Hyperventilation with hypoxia.
- *Stage 3*: A false-normal PCO_2 which is an extremely serious sign of respiratory muscle fatigue.
- *Stage 4*: Hypoxemia and a high PCO_2, which occurs with respiratory failure and needs ventilatory support.

- **Minimal alveolar concentration**: The lowest concentration of the anesthetic in pulmonary alveoli needed to produce immobility in response to a painful stimulus in 50% individuals.
- **Second gas effect**: During induction of general anesthesia, when a large volume of a gas (e.g. nitrous oxide) is taken up from alveoli into pulmonary capillary blood, the concentration of gases remaining in the alveoli is increased. This results in effects known as the "concentration effect" and the second gas effect where the gas mixture will be sucked in independent of ventilatory exchange; thus gas flow will be higher than tidal volume.

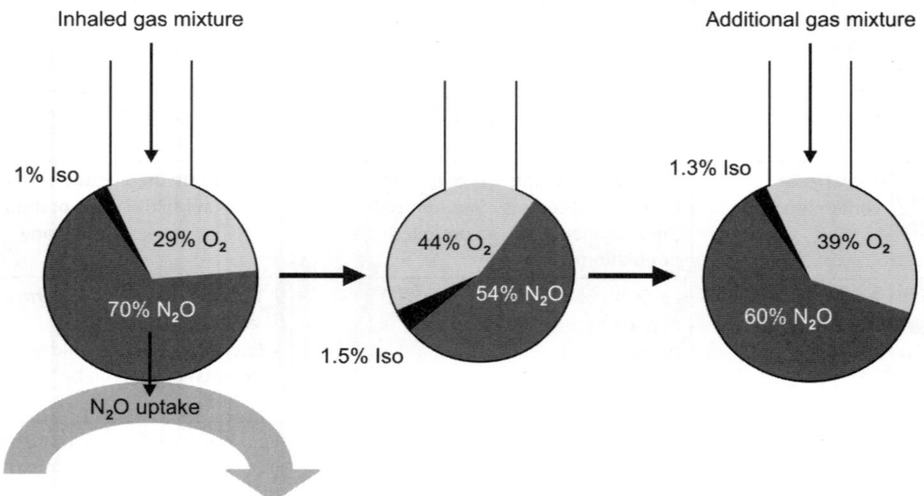

Fig. 1.7: The concept of second gas effect
Source: Congnecker DE, Brown DL, Newman MF, Zapol WM. Anesthesiology, 2nd edn. *www.accessanesthesiology.com*

- **Diffusion hypoxia**: During discontinuation of N_2O after prolonged anesthesia the reverse of second gas effect occurs leading to dilution of the alveolar air and finally PP of oxygen is reduced, this resulting hypoxia is called diffusion hypoxia.
- **Epilepsy**: The term 'epilepsy' denotes any disorder characterized by recurrent unprovoked seizures (CMDT 2017). Seizure is defined as a paroxysmal event due to abnormal excessive or synchronous neuronal activity in the brain.
- **Status epilepticus**: It refers to continuous seizures or repetitive, discrete seizures with impaired consciousness in the inter-ictal period. The duration of seizure activity sufficient to meet the definition of status epilepticus has traditionally been specified as 15–30.
- **Hypertensive urgency**: SBP>220 mm Hg or DBP>120 mm Hg without overt signs of end organ damage.
- **Hypertensive emergency**: SBP>220 mm Hg or DBP>120 mm Hg with active evidence of end organ damage.

- **Diuretics (Natriuretics)**: These are drugs which cause a net loss of Na^+ and water in urine.
- **Free water clearance**: It is defined as the volume of urine excreted per unit time in excess of that required to excrete the contained solute isosmotically with plasma.
  - *Positive free water clearance*: Urine is dilute wrt plasma.
  - *Negative free water clearance*: Urine is concentrated wrt plasma.
  - *Zero free water clearance*: Isosmotic with plasma.
- **Hematinics**: These are substances required in the formation of blood and are used for the treatment of anemias, e.g. iron, folic acid, etc.
  Unconventional hematinics: Erythropoietin, lithium, thyroxine.
- **Laxatives and purgatives**: Chemical agents that promote evacuation of bowel and are primarily used to treat constipation or when loose stools are desirable. Based on their intensity of action they are classified as:
  - *Laxatives or aperients*: Milder action and thus lead to elimination of soft but formed stools.
  - *Purgatives or cathartics*: Stronger action resulting in fluid evacuation.
- **Chelating agents**: These are drugs that can form ring structures within their molecule with metallic ions thus producing stable, non-toxic and easily excretable complexes.
  Orally active iron chelator- deferiprone, deferasirox.
- **Vaccine/sera**: These are biological products which act by reinforcing the immunological defence of the body against foreign agents mostly infective organisms or their toxins.
- **Toxoid**: A toxoid is a bacterial toxin (usually an exotoxin) whose toxicity has been inactivated or suppressed, while other properties, typically immunogenicity, are maintained. Thus, when used during vaccination, an immune response is mounted and immunological memory is formed against the molecular markers of the toxoid without resulting in toxin-induced illness.
- **Antisera**: These are purified and concentrated preparations of serum of horses actively immunized against a specific antigen.
- **Antiseptic and disinfectant**: These two terms connote an agent which inhibits or kills microbes on contact. Conventionally, agents used on living surfaces are called antiseptics while those used on inanimate objects are called disinfectants.
- **Irritant**: These are drugs that stimulate sensory nerve endings and induce inflammation at the site of application.
- **Counter irritant**: Certain irritants also produce a remote effect which tends to relieve pain and inflammation in deeper organs, e. g. clove oil, methyl salicylate.
- **Vesicant**: Stronger irritants which in addition increase capillary permeability and cause collection of fluid under the epidermis forming vesicles, e. g. vancomycin.
- **Rubefacient**: Irritants which cause local hyperemia with little sensory competent, e. g. capsaicin.
- **Emollient**: These are bland oily substances which soothe and soften skin, e.g. olive oil.
- **Demulcent**: Inert substances which soothe inflamed or denuded mucosa or skin by preventing contact with air/irritants in the surroundings, e. g. glycyrrhiza, methylcellulose
- **Astringent**: These are substances that precipitate proteins, but do not penetrate cells thus affecting the superficial layer only, e. g. tannic acid.

- **Adsorbents and protectives**: These are finely powdered, inert and insoluble solids capable of binding to their surface (adsorbing) noxious and irritant substances, e. g. talc, aloe vera.
- **Ointment**: It is a semisolid preparation containing medicinal ingredients for external use only on skin/mucous membranes.

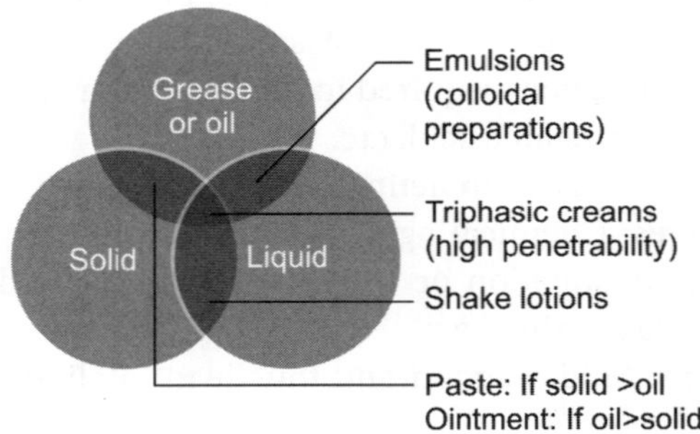

Fig. 1.8: Venn diagram showing different types of topical applications and their composition

- **FTU (Fingertip unit)**: It is the unit of application of ointments. 1 FTU ~ 0.5 g/area of 2 palms. 20 FTU ~ whole body.
- **Antibiotic**: These are substances produced by microorganisms, which selectively suppress the growth of or kill other microorganisms at very low concentrations.
- **Antimicrobial agent (AMA)**: This is a common term to designate both synthetic and naturally derived drugs that attenuate microorganisms.
  Thus, all antibiotics are also antimicrobials but the reverse is not true. For example, silver
- **Anticancer**: These are drugs that either kill cancer cells or modify their growth.
- **DOTS**: Directly observed treatment short-course (DOTS) is a domiciliary treatment strategy to ensure cure of TB by providing most effective regimen of medicines and also confirming that medicines are taken.
- **Monoresistance TB**: Resistance to one 1st line anti-TB drug only.
- **Polydrug resistance TB**: Resistance to more than one 1st line anti-TB drug (other than INH and rifampicin).
- **Multidrug resistance TB**: Resistance to at least both INH and rifampicin (i.e. may have resistance of other 1st line drugs).
- **Extensive drug resistance TB**: Resistance to any fluoroquinolone and at least one of the 2nd line injectable drugs (capreomycin, amikacin, kanamycin); in addition to multidrug resistance.
- **MIC**: Minimum inhibitory concentration (MIC) is the lowest concentration of an antibiotic which prevents visible growth of a bacterium after 24 hrs incubation in micro-well culture plates using serial dilutions of the antibiotic.
- **MBC**: Minimum bactericidal concentration (MBC) of an antibiotic is determined by subculturing from tubes with no visible growth denotes killing of the organism.
  - *Bactericidal antibiotic*: Small difference between MIC and MBC.
  - *Bacteriostatic antibiotic*: Large difference between MIC and MBC.

- **Post-antibiotic effect**: The lag period in growth resumption when after a brief exposure to an antibiotic, the organism is placed in an antibiotic free medium; it starts multiplying again, is called post-antibiotic effect. It depends on the antibiotic as well as the organism.

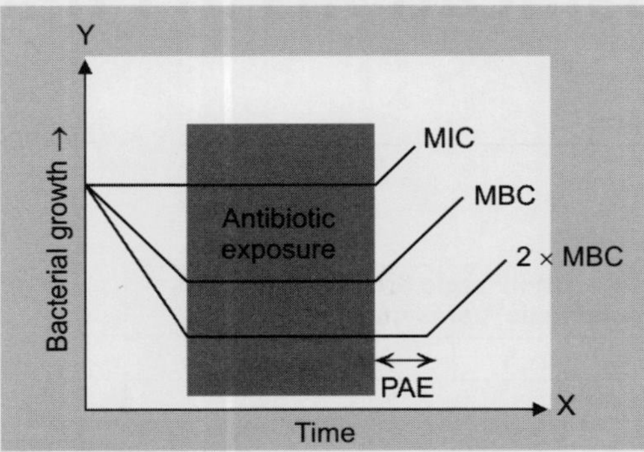

Fig. 1.9: The concept of minimum inhibitory concentration, minimum bactericidal concentration and post-antibiotic effect

- **Break point concentration**: It is defined as the concentration of antibiotic that demarcates between sensitive and resistant bacteria.

CHAPTER 2

Classifications in Pharmacology

Avishek Layek, Dyuti Deepta Rano

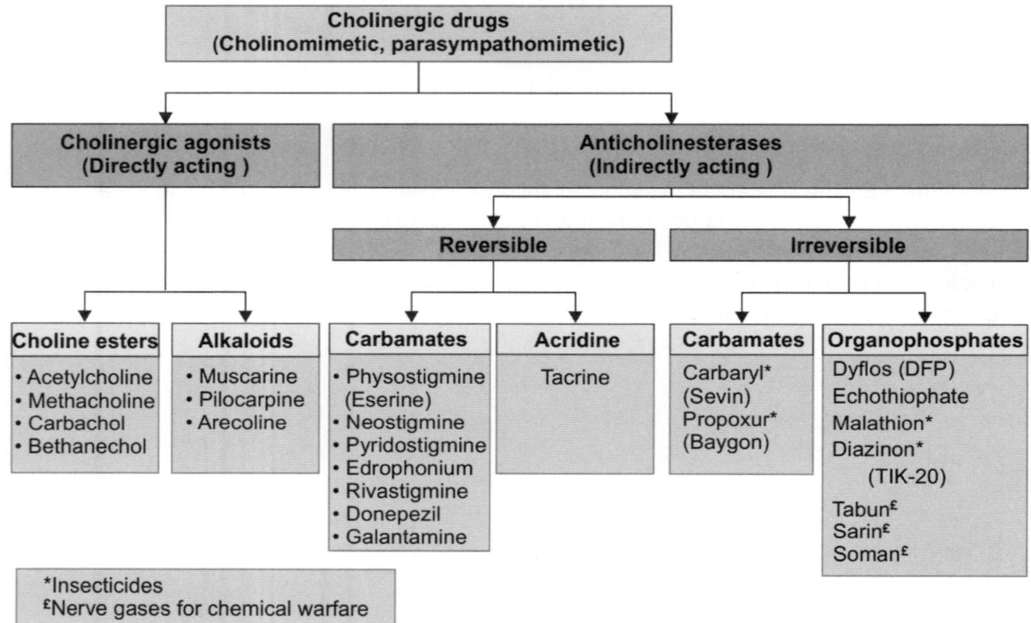

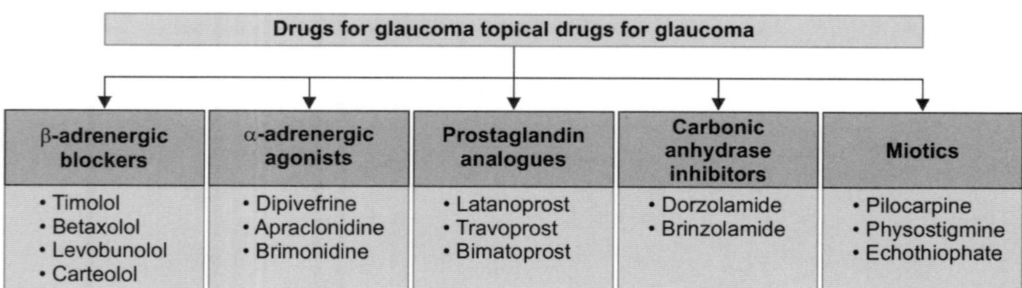

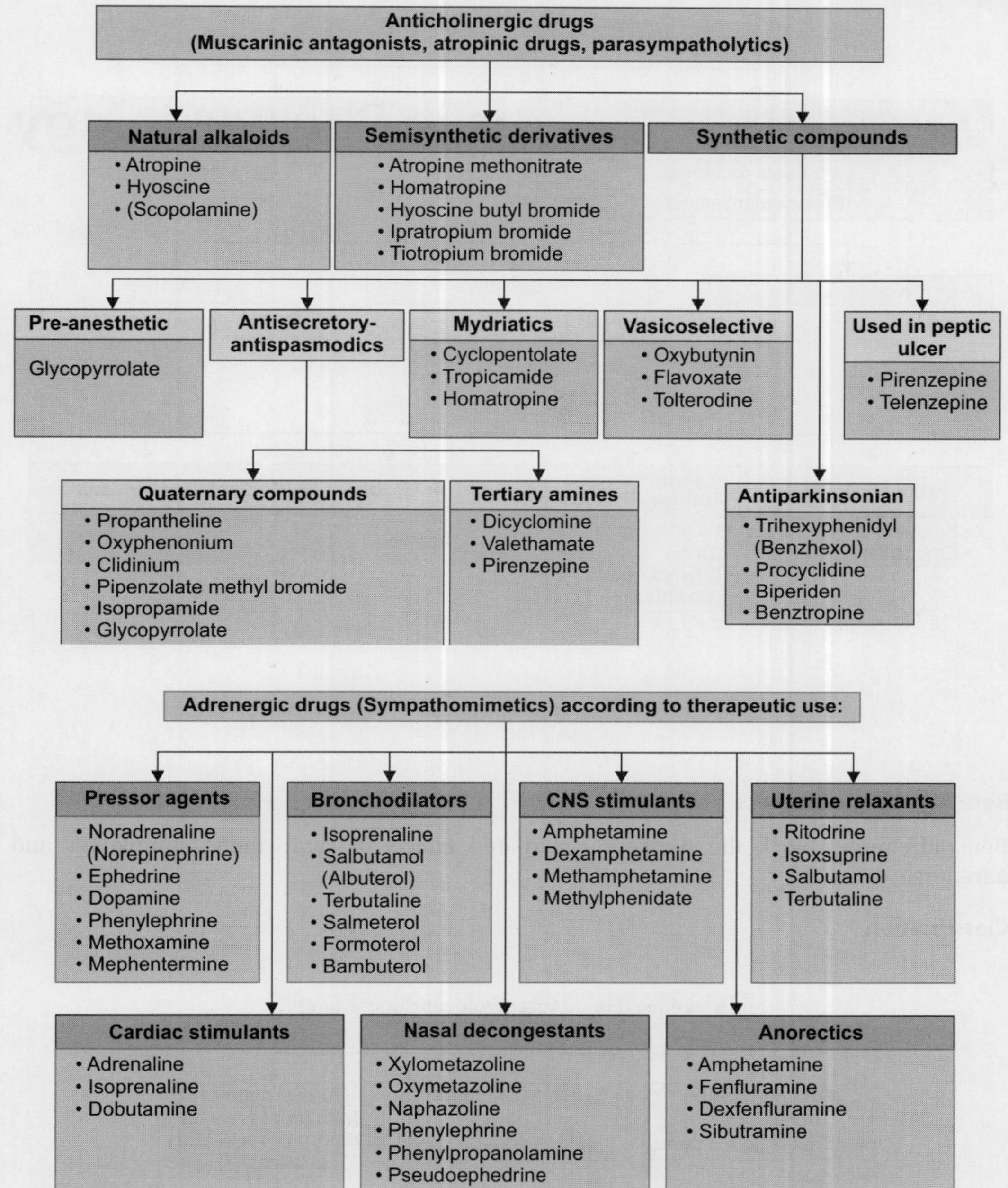

Adrenergic drugs: According to chemical structure

1. Catecholamines: Adrenaline, Noradrenaline, Dopamine, Dobutamine
2. Non-catecholamines: Tyramine, Ephedrine, Salbutamol, Amphetamine

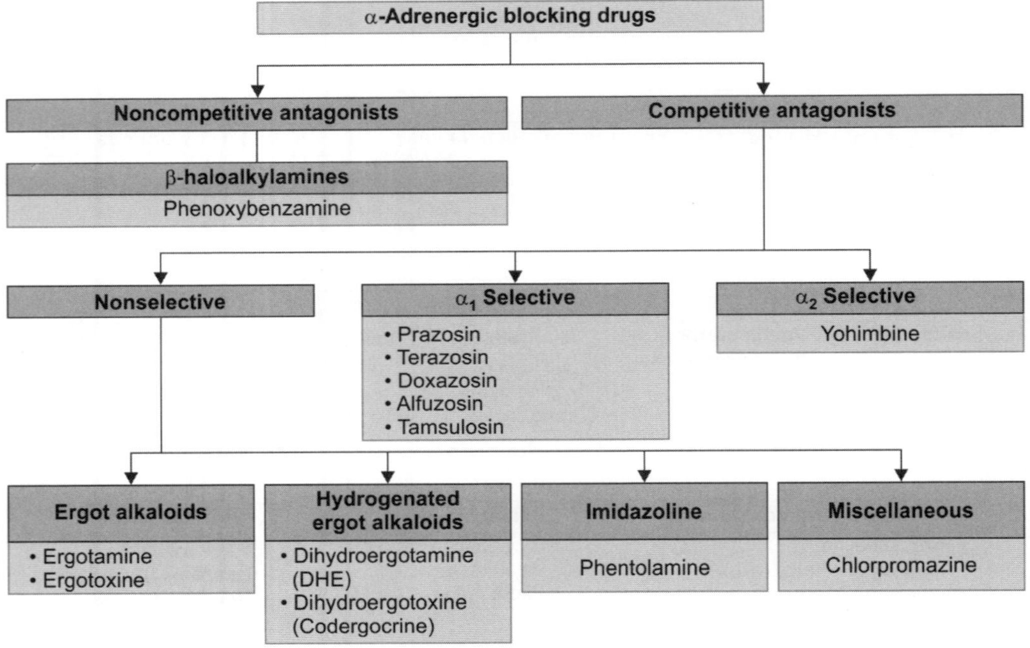

Beta Adrenergic Blockers

Beta adrenergic block the β-receptor-mediated effects of sympathetic stimulation and adrenergic drugs.

Classification

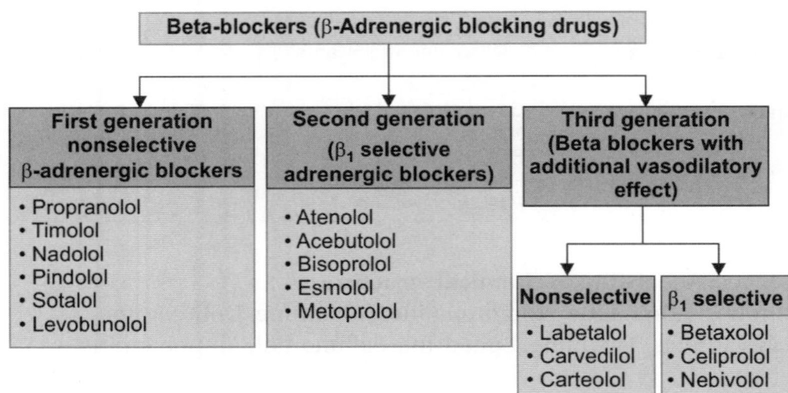

Drugs for migraine

- **To acute attacks**
  - **Simple analgesics**
    - Paracetamol
    - Aspirin
    - Metamizol
    - Codeine
  - **NSAIDs**
    - Ibuprofen
    - Naproxen
    - Diclofenac
    - Mephenamic acid
  - **Antiemetics**
    - Metoclopramide
    - Domperidone
    - Prochlorperazine
    - Promethazine
  - **Ergot alkaloids**
    - Ergotamine
    - Dihydroergotamine (DHE)
  - **Selective 5-HT$_{ID/IB}$ agonists**
    - Sumatriptan
    - Rizatriptan
    - Naratriptan
    - Zolmitriptan
    - Frovatriptan
- **For prophylaxis**
  - Propranolol (other β-blockers)
  - Amitriptyline (other TCAs)
  - Flunarizine
  - Valproic acid
  - Gabapentin
  - Topiramate
  - Cyproheptadine

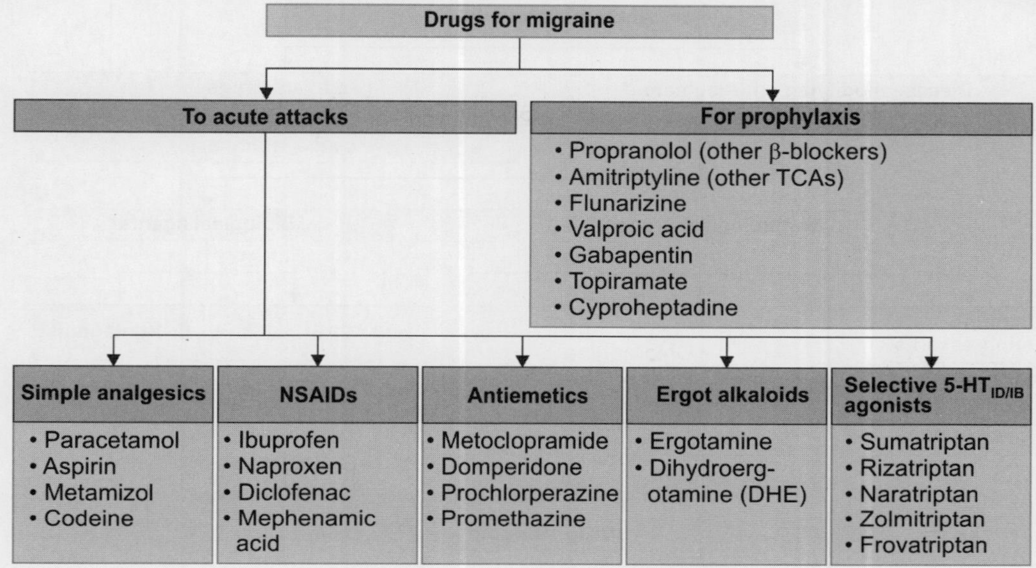

Nonsteroidal anti-inflammatory drugs/ antipyretic-analgesics

- **Nonselective COX inhibitors**
  - **Salicylates**
    - Aspirin
  - **Propionic acid derivatives**
    - Ibuprofen
    - Naproxen
    - Ketoprofen
    - Flurbiprofen
  - **Fenamate**
    - Mefenamic acid
  - **Enolic acid derivatives**
    - Piroxicam
    - Tenoxicam
  - **Acetic acid derivatives**
    - Ketorolac
    - Indomethacin
    - Nabumetone
  - **Pyrazolone derivatives**
    - Phenylbutazone
    - Oxyphenbutazone
- **Preferential COX-2 inhibitors**
  - Nimesulide
  - Diclofenac
  - Aceclofenac
  - Meloxicam
  - Etodolac
- **Selective COX-2 inhibitors**
  - Celecoxib
  - Etoricoxib
  - Parecoxib
- **Analgesic-antipyretics with poor anti-inflammatory action**
  - **Para-aminophenol derivative**
    - Acetaminophen (also blocks cox-3)
  - **Pyrazolone derivatives**
    - Metamizol (Dipyrone)
    - Propyphenazone (PPPZ)
  - **Benzoxazocine derivative (BZ x Z)**
    - Nefopam

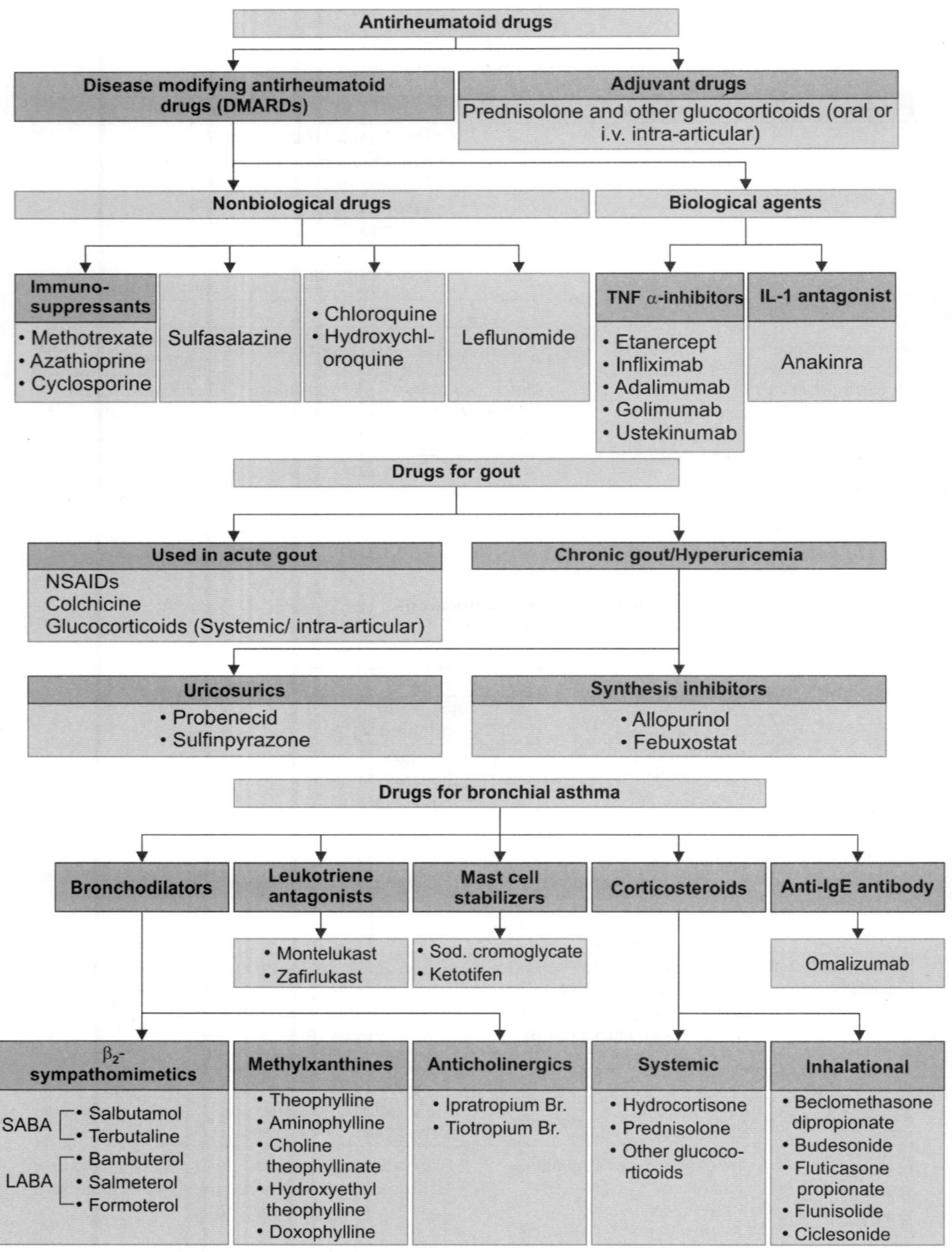

Abbreviations: SABA, short acting β-agonists; LABA, long acting β-agonists

Thyroid inhibitors

- **Others**
  - Lithium
  - Amiodarone
  - PAS
  - Phneobarbitone
- **Inhibit hormone synthesis**
  - (Antithyroid drugs)
  - Propylthiouracil
  - Methimazole
  - Carbimazole
- **Inhibit iodide trapping**
  - (Ionic inhibitors)
  - Thiocyanates (–SCN)
  - Perchlorates (–ClO_4)
  - Nitrates (–NO_3)
- **Inhibit hormone release**
  - Iodine
  - Iodides of Na, K
  - Organic iodide
- **Destroy thyroid tissue**
  - Radioactive iodine ^{131}I
- **Goitrogens**
  - Bressica vegetables

Insulins

- **Rapid acting**
  - (Insulin analogues)
  - Insulin lispro
  - Insulin aspart
  - Insulin glulisine
- **Short acting**
  - Regular (soluble) insulin
- **Intermediate acting**
  - Insulin zinc suspension (Lente insulin)
  - Neutral protamine hagedorn (NPH) or isophane insulin
- **Long acting**
  - (Insulin analogues)
  - Insulin glargine
  - Insulin detemir
  - Insulin degludec

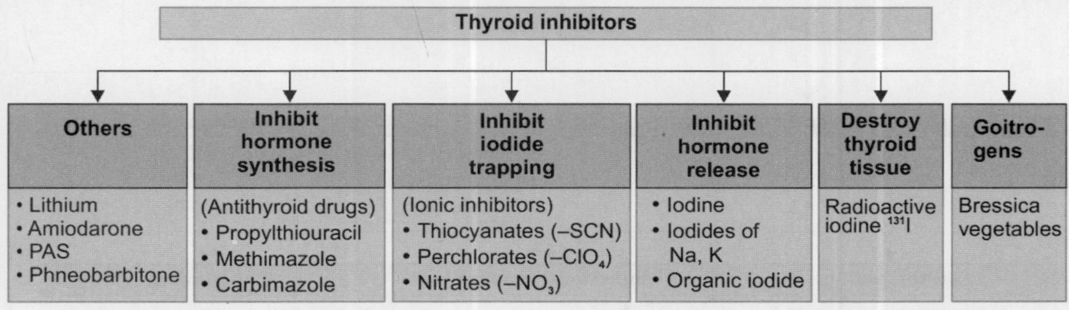

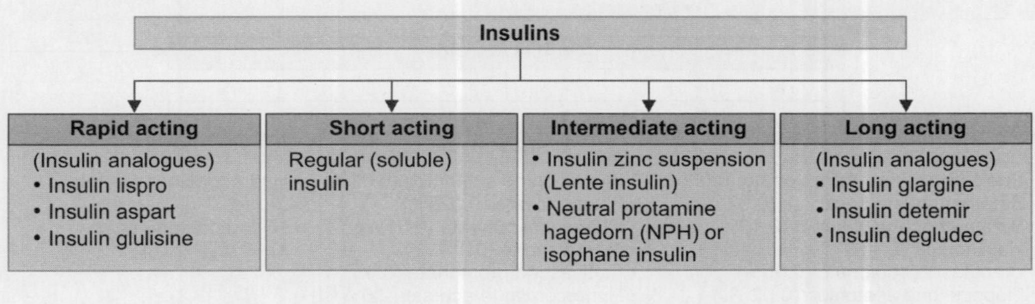

Skeletal muscle relaxants

- **Peripherally acting**
  - **Neuromuscular blocking agents**
    - **Nondepolarizing (competitive) blockers**
      - **Long acting**
        - d-tubocurarine
        - Pancuronium
        - Doxacurium
        - Pipecuronium
      - **Intermediate acting**
        - Vecuronium
        - Atracurium
        - Cisatracurium
        - Rocuronium
        - Rapacuronium
      - **Short acting**
        - Mivacurium
    - **Depolarizing blockers**
      - Succinyl choline (suxamethonium)
      - Decamethonium
  - **Directly acting agents**
    - Dantrolene sodium
    - Quinine
- **Centrally acting**
  - **Mephenesin congeners**
    - Carisoprodol
    - Chlorzoxazone
    - Chlormezanone
    - Methocarbamol
  - **Benzodiazepines**
    - Diazepam, etc.
  - **GABA mimetic**
    - Baclofen
    - Thiocolchicoside
  - **Central α_2-agonist**
    - Tizanidine

Corticosteroids

- **Glucocorticoids**
  - **Short acting**
    - Hydrocortisone (Cortisol)
  - **Intermediate acting**
    - Prednisolone
    - Methyl prednisolone
    - Triamcinolone
    - Deflazacort
  - **Long acting**
    - Dexamethasone
    - Betamethasone
- **Mineralocorticoids**
  - Desoxycorticosterone acetate (DOCA)
  - Fludrocortisone
  - Aldosterone
- **Topical steroids**
  - **Potent**
    - Beclomethasone dipropionate (0.025%)
    - Betamethasone benzoate (0.025%)
    - Betamethasone valerate (0.12%)
    - Halcinonide (0.1%)
    - Clobetasol propionate (0.05%)
    - Fluocinolone acetonide (0.025%)
    - Fluocortolone (0.5%)
    - Triamcinolone acetonide (0.1%)
    - Dexamethasone sod. phos. (0.1%)
  - **Moderately potent**
    - Fluocinolone acetonide (0.01%)
    - Fluocortolone (0.025%)
    - Clobetasol butyrate (0.05%)
    - Mometasone (0.1%)
    - Fluticasone propionate (0.05%)
    - Hydrocortisone acetate (2.5%)
  - **Mild**
    - Hydrocortisone acetate (0.1–1.0%)
    - Hydrocortisone butyrate (0.001%)

General anesthetics

- **Inhalational**
  - **Gas**
    - Nitrous oxide
  - **Volatile liquids**
    - Ether
    - Halothane
    - Isoflurane
    - Desflurane
    - Sevoflurane
- **Intravenous**
  - **Fast acting drugs**
    - Thiopentone sodium
    - Methohexitone sodium
    - Propofol
    - Etomidate
  - **Slower acting drugs**
    - **Benzodiazepines**
      - Diazepam
      - Lorazepam
      - Midazolam
    - **Dissociative anesthetic**
      - Ketamine
    - **Opioid analgesic**
      - Fentanyl

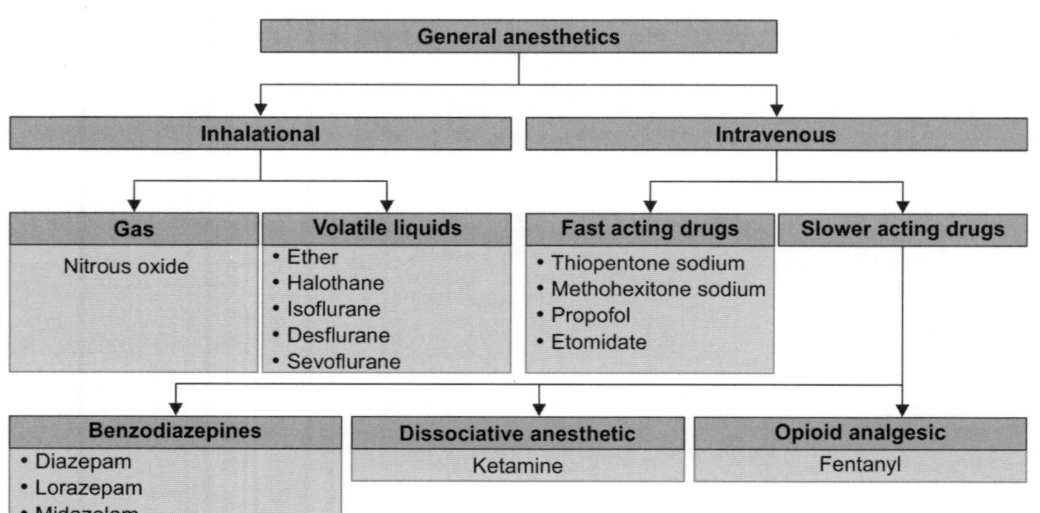

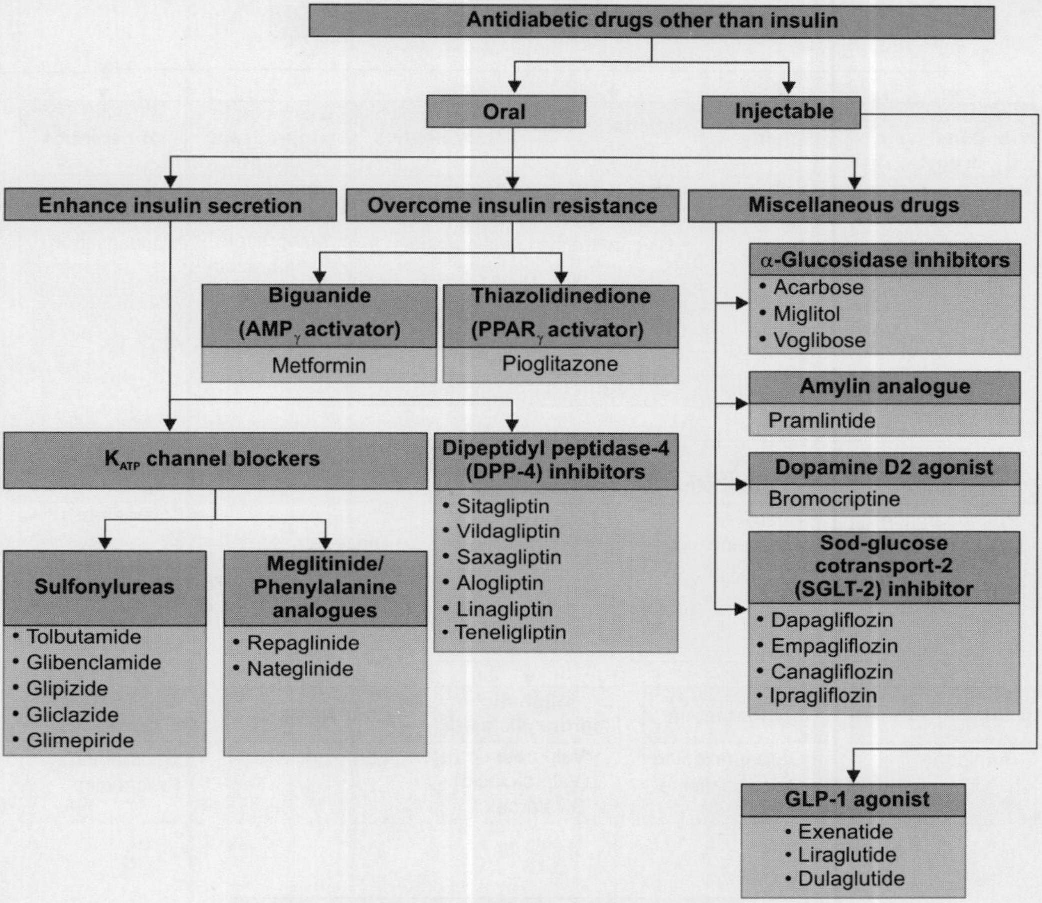

Antidiabetic drugs other than insulin

- **Oral**
  - **Enhance insulin secretion**
    - **K_{ATP} channel blockers**
      - **Sulfonylureas**
        - Tolbutamide
        - Glibenclamide
        - Glipizide
        - Gliclazide
        - Glimepiride
      - **Meglitinide/Phenylalanine analogues**
        - Repaglinide
        - Nateglinide
    - **Dipeptidyl peptidase-4 (DPP-4) inhibitors**
      - Sitagliptin
      - Vildagliptin
      - Saxagliptin
      - Alogliptin
      - Linagliptin
      - Teneligliptin
  - **Overcome insulin resistance**
    - **Biguanide (AMP_{γ} activator)**: Metformin
    - **Thiazolidinedione ($PPAR_{\gamma}$ activator)**: Pioglitazone
  - **Miscellaneous drugs**
    - **α-Glucosidase inhibitors**
      - Acarbose
      - Miglitol
      - Voglibose
    - **Amylin analogue**: Pramlintide
    - **Dopamine D2 agonist**: Bromocriptine
    - **Sod-glucose cotransport-2 (SGLT-2) inhibitor**
      - Dapagliflozin
      - Empagliflozin
      - Canagliflozin
      - Ipragliflozin
- **Injectable**
  - **GLP-1 agonist**
    - Exenatide
    - Liraglutide
    - Dulaglutide

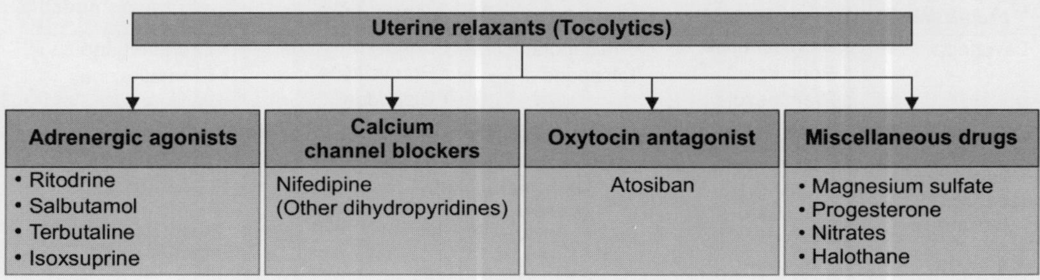

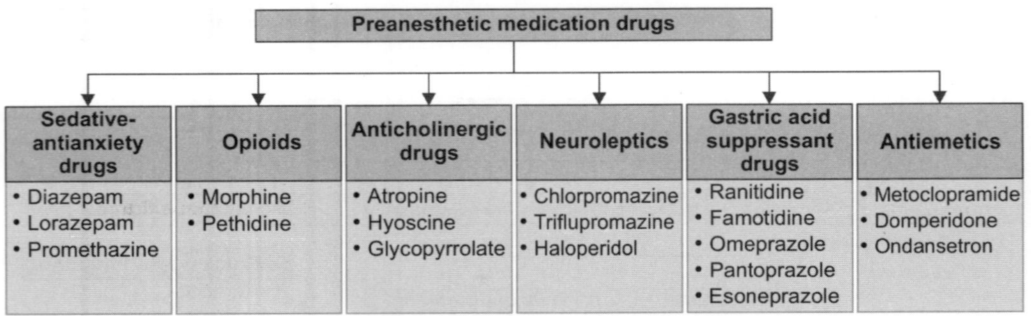
Preanesthetic medication drugs
Sedative-antianxiety drugs
• Diazepam
• Lorazepam
• Promethazine
Opioids
• Morphine
• Pethidine
Anticholinergic drugs
• Atropine
• Hyoscine
• Glycopyrrolate
Neuroleptics
• Chlorpromazine
• Triflupromazine
• Haloperidol
Gastric acid suppressant drugs
• Ranitidine
• Famotidine
• Omeprazole
• Pantoprazole
• Esoneprazole
Antiemetics
• Metoclopramide
• Domperidone
• Ondansetron

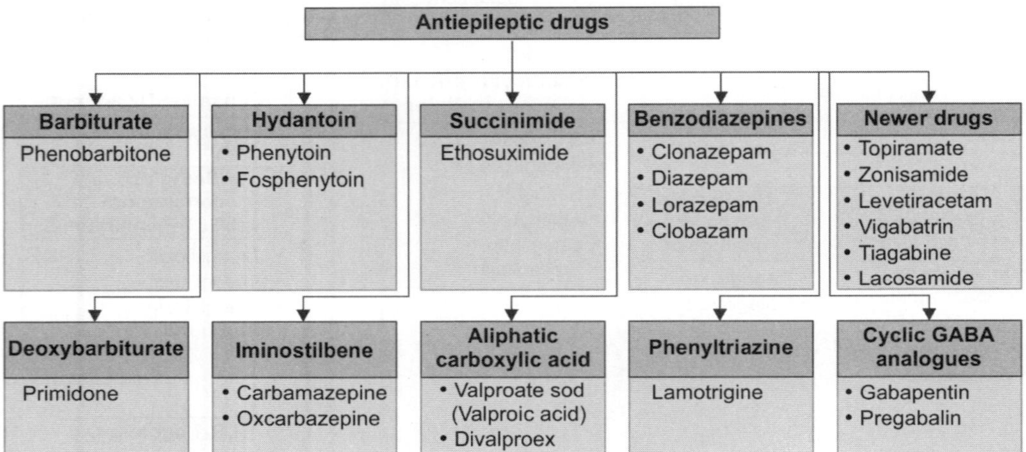
Antiepileptic drugs
Barbiturate
Phenobarbitone
Hydantoin
• Phenytoin
• Fosphenytoin
Succinimide
Ethosuximide
Benzodiazepines
• Clonazepam
• Diazepam
• Lorazepam
• Clobazam
Newer drugs
• Topiramate
• Zonisamide
• Levetiracetam
• Vigabatrin
• Tiagabine
• Lacosamide
Deoxybarbiturate
Primidone
Iminostilbene
• Carbamazepine
• Oxcarbazepine
Aliphatic carboxylic acid
• Valproate sod (Valproic acid)
• Divalproex
Phenyltriazine
Lamotrigine
Cyclic GABA analogues
• Gabapentin
• Pregabalin

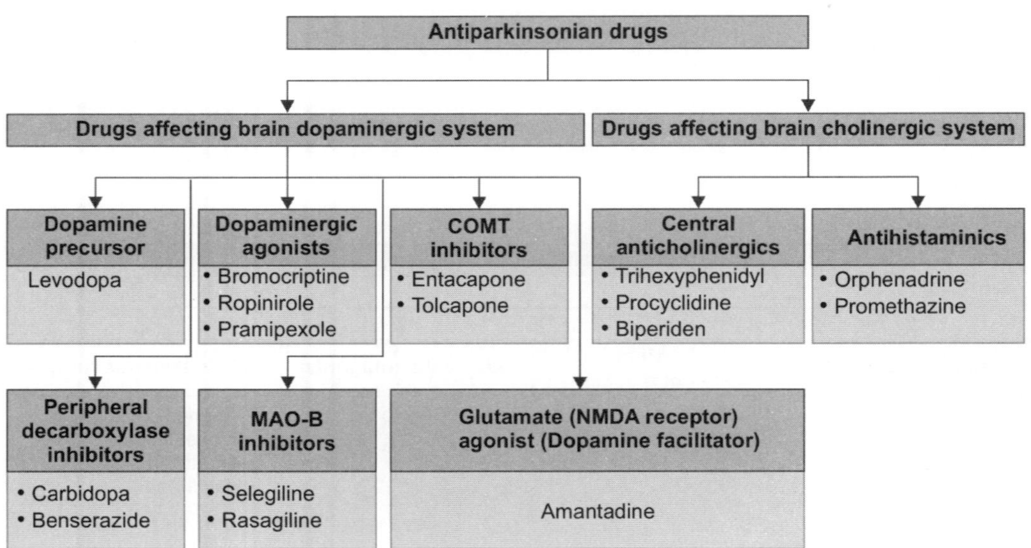
Antiparkinsonian drugs
Drugs affecting brain dopaminergic system
Drugs affecting brain cholinergic system
Dopamine precursor
Levodopa
Dopaminergic agonists
• Bromocriptine
• Ropinirole
• Pramipexole
COMT inhibitors
• Entacapone
• Tolcapone
Central anticholinergics
• Trihexyphenidyl
• Procyclidine
• Biperiden
Antihistaminics
• Orphenadrine
• Promethazine
Peripheral decarboxylase inhibitors
• Carbidopa
• Benserazide
MAO-B inhibitors
• Selegiline
• Rasagiline
Glutamate (NMDA receptor) agonist (Dopamine facilitator)
Amantadine

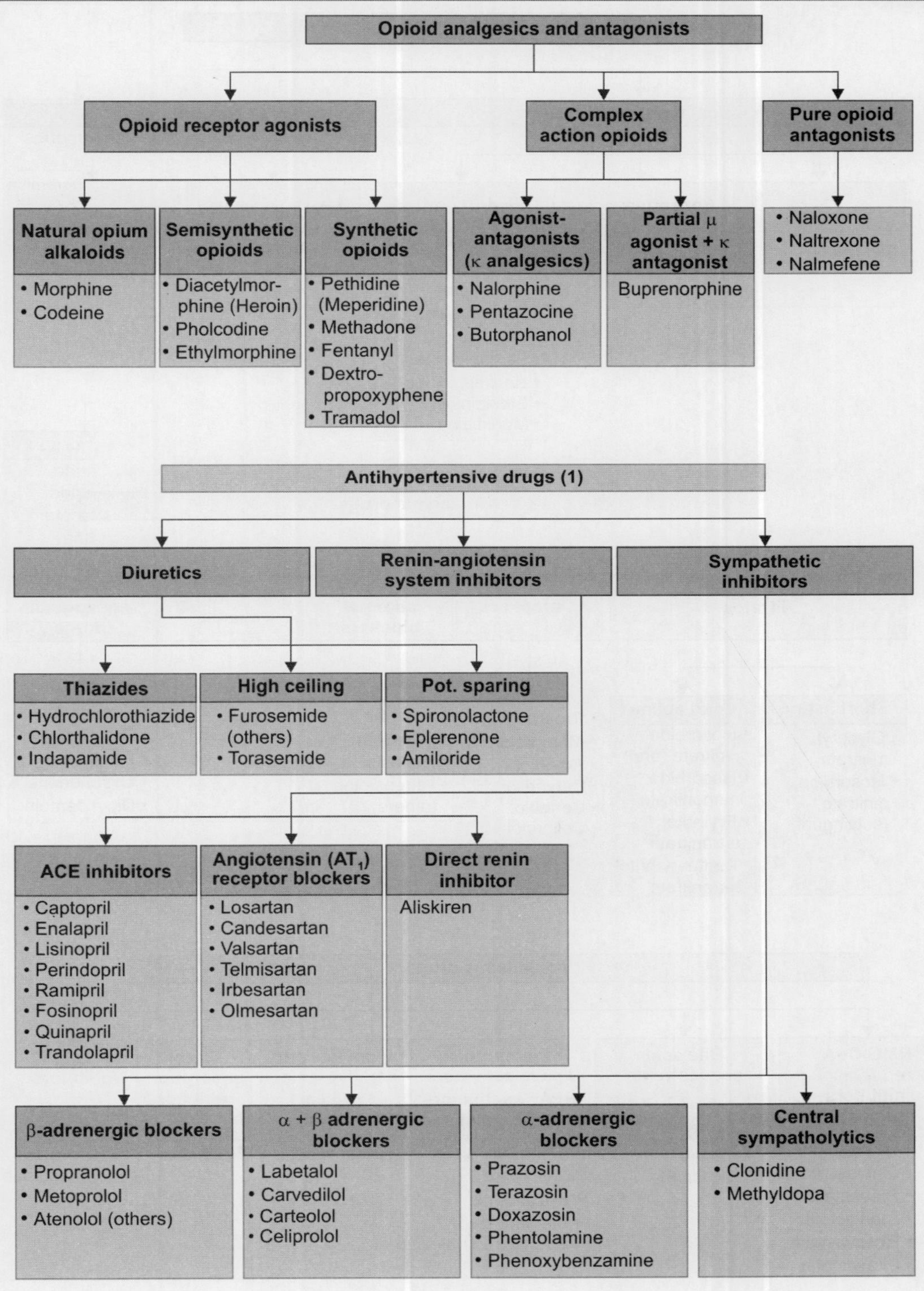
Opioid analgesics and antagonists
Opioid receptor agonists
Complex action opioids
Pure opioid antagonists
Natural opium alkaloids
• Morphine
• Codeine
Semisynthetic opioids
• Diacetylmorphine (Heroin)
• Pholcodine
• Ethylmorphine
Synthetic opioids
• Pethidine (Meperidine)
• Methadone
• Fentanyl
• Dextro-propoxyphene
• Tramadol
Agonist-antagonists (κ analgesics)
• Nalorphine
• Pentazocine
• Butorphanol
Partial μ agonist + κ antagonist
Buprenorphine
• Naloxone
• Naltrexone
• Nalmefene
Antihypertensive drugs (1)
Diuretics
Renin-angiotensin system inhibitors
Sympathetic inhibitors
Thiazides
• Hydrochlorothiazide
• Chlorthalidone
• Indapamide
High ceiling
• Furosemide (others)
• Torasemide
Pot. sparing
• Spironolactone
• Eplerenone
• Amiloride
ACE inhibitors
• Captopril
• Enalapril
• Lisinopril
• Perindopril
• Ramipril
• Fosinopril
• Quinapril
• Trandolapril
Angiotensin (AT1) receptor blockers
• Losartan
• Candesartan
• Valsartan
• Telmisartan
• Irbesartan
• Olmesartan
Direct renin inhibitor
Aliskiren
β-adrenergic blockers
• Propranolol
• Metoprolol
• Atenolol (others)
α + β adrenergic blockers
• Labetalol
• Carvedilol
• Carteolol
• Celiprolol
α-adrenergic blockers
• Prazosin
• Terazosin
• Doxazosin
• Phentolamine
• Phenoxybenzamine
Central sympatholytics
• Clonidine
• Methyldopa

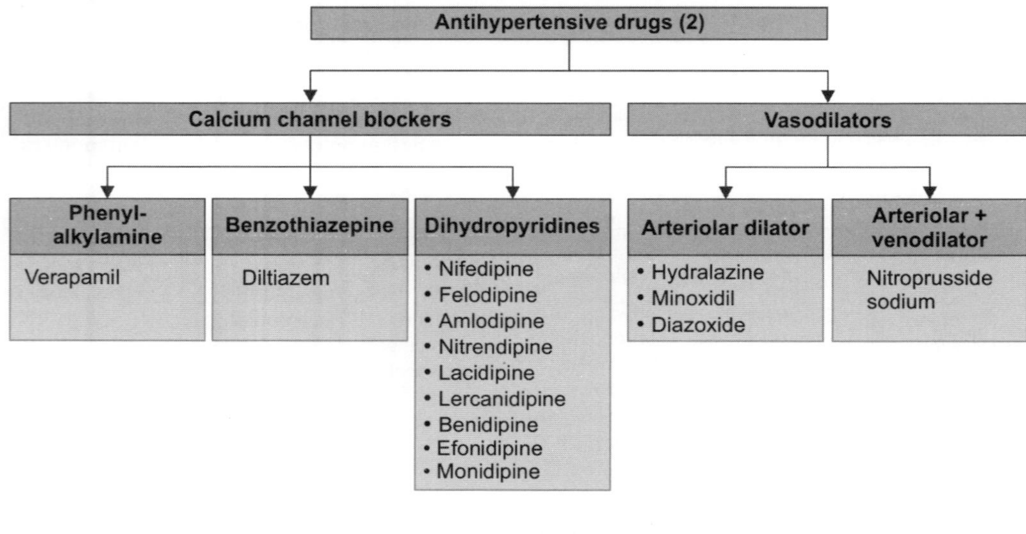
Antihypertensive drugs (2)
Calcium channel blockers
Vasodilators
Phenyl-alkylamine
Benzothiazepine
Dihydropyridines
Arteriolar dilator
Arteriolar + venodilator
Verapamil
Diltiazem
• Nifedipine
• Felodipine
• Amlodipine
• Nitrendipine
• Lacidipine
• Lercanidipine
• Benidipine
• Efonidipine
• Monidipine
• Hydralazine
• Minoxidil
• Diazoxide
Nitroprusside sodium

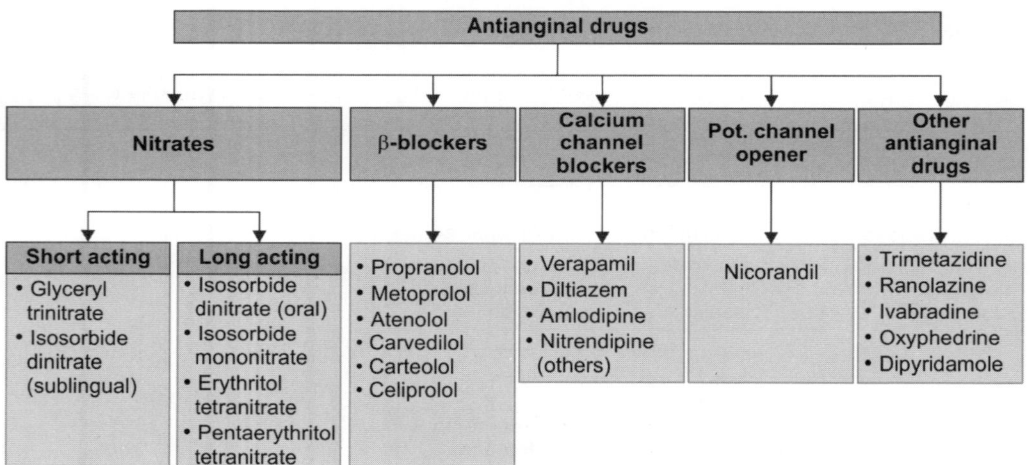
Antianginal drugs
Nitrates
β-blockers
Calcium channel blockers
Pot. channel opener
Other antianginal drugs
Short acting
Long acting
• Glyceryl trinitrate
• Isosorbide dinitrate (sublingual)
• Isosorbide dinitrate (oral)
• Isosorbide mononitrate
• Erythritol tetranitrate
• Pentaerythritol tetranitrate
• Propranolol
• Metoprolol
• Atenolol
• Carvedilol
• Carteolol
• Celiprolol
• Verapamil
• Diltiazem
• Amlodipine
• Nitrendipine (others)
Nicorandil
• Trimetazidine
• Ranolazine
• Ivabradine
• Oxyphedrine
• Dipyridamole

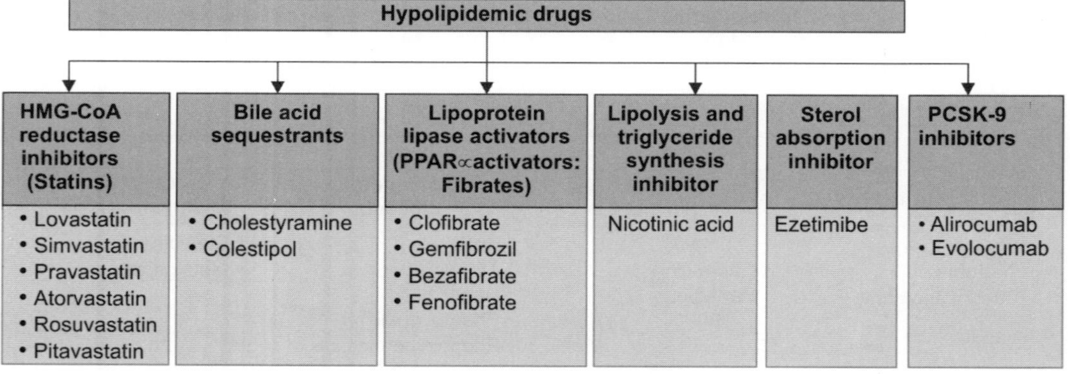
Hypolipidemic drugs
HMG-CoA reductase inhibitors (Statins)
Bile acid sequestrants
Lipoprotein lipase activators (PPARα activators: Fibrates)
Lipolysis and triglyceride synthesis inhibitor
Sterol absorption inhibitor
PCSK-9 inhibitors
• Lovastatin
• Simvastatin
• Pravastatin
• Atorvastatin
• Rosuvastatin
• Pitavastatin
• Cholestyramine
• Colestipol
• Clofibrate
• Gemfibrozil
• Bezafibrate
• Fenofibrate
Nicotinic acid
Ezetimibe
• Alirocumab
• Evolocumab

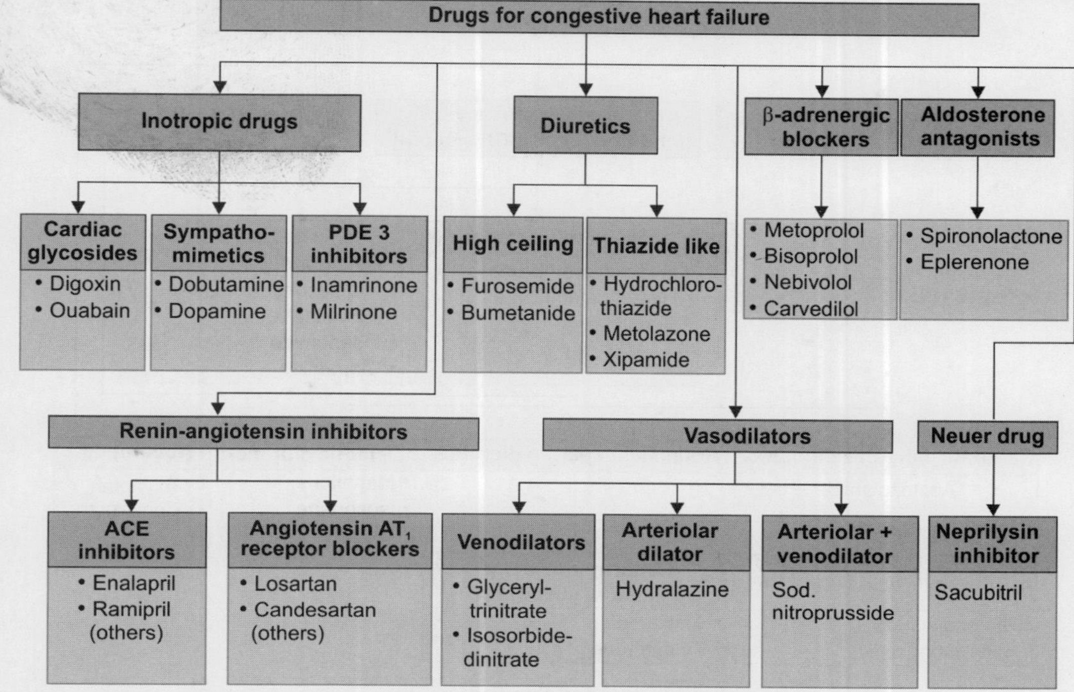

Abbreviations: PDE, phosphodiesterase; ACE, angiotensin converting enzyme

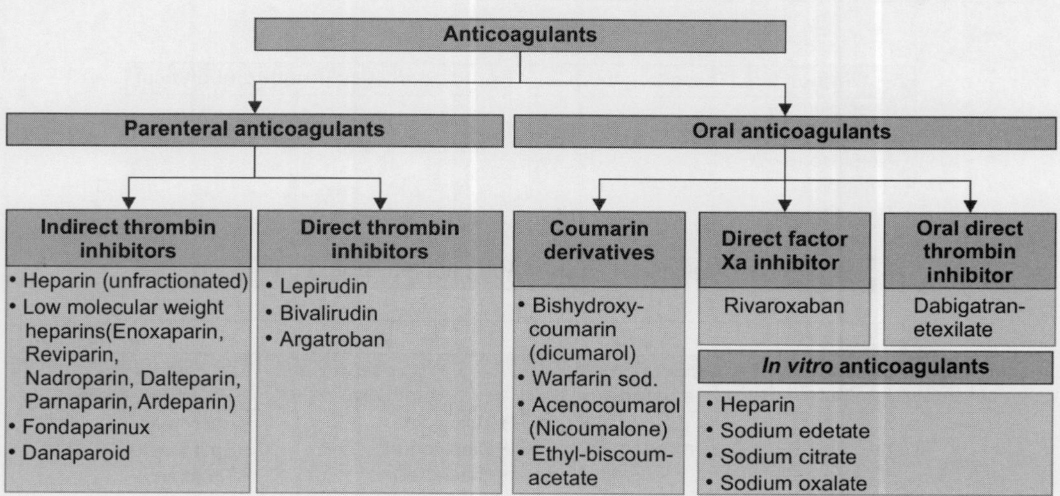

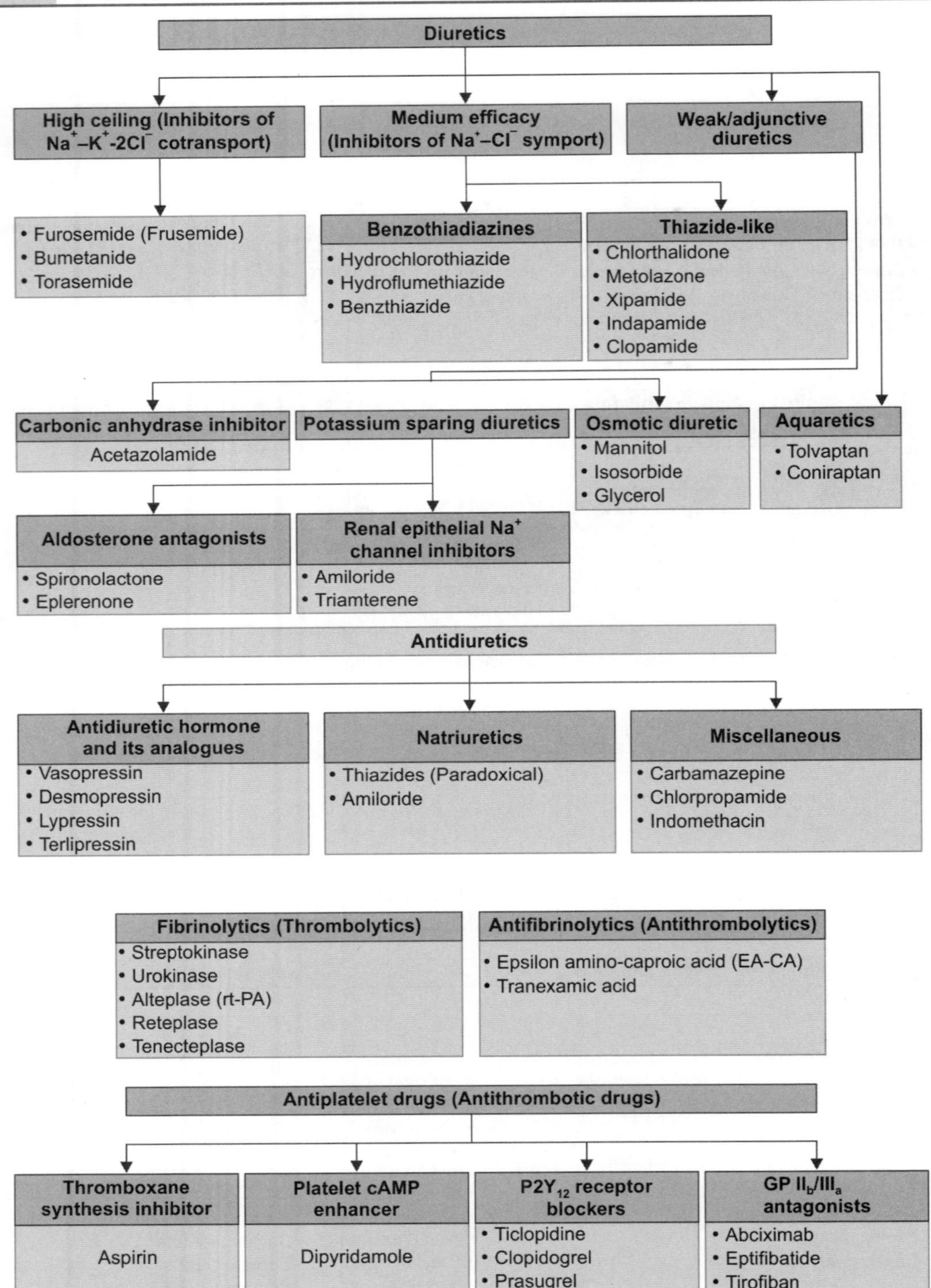

Diuretics
High ceiling (Inhibitors of Na^+–K^+-2Cl^- cotransport)
• Furosemide (Frusemide)
• Bumetanide
• Torasemide
Medium efficacy (Inhibitors of Na^+–Cl^- symport)
Benzothiadiazines
• Hydrochlorothiazide
• Hydroflumethiazide
• Benzthiazide
Thiazide-like
• Chlorthalidone
• Metolazone
• Xipamide
• Indapamide
• Clopamide
Weak/adjunctive diuretics
Carbonic anhydrase inhibitor
Acetazolamide
Potassium sparing diuretics
Aldosterone antagonists
• Spironolactone
• Eplerenone
Renal epithelial Na^+ channel inhibitors
• Amiloride
• Triamterene
Osmotic diuretic
• Mannitol
• Isosorbide
• Glycerol
Aquaretics
• Tolvaptan
• Coniraptan
Antidiuretics
Antidiuretic hormone and its analogues
• Vasopressin
• Desmopressin
• Lypressin
• Terlipressin
Natriuretics
• Thiazides (Paradoxical)
• Amiloride
Miscellaneous
• Carbamazepine
• Chlorpropamide
• Indomethacin
Fibrinolytics (Thrombolytics)
• Streptokinase
• Urokinase
• Alteplase (rt-PA)
• Reteplase
• Tenecteplase
Antifibrinolytics (Antithrombolytics)
• Epsilon amino-caproic acid (EA-CA)
• Tranexamic acid
Antiplatelet drugs (Antithrombotic drugs)
Thromboxane synthesis inhibitor
Aspirin
Platelet cAMP enhancer
Dipyridamole
$P2Y_{12}$ receptor blockers
• Ticlopidine
• Clopidogrel
• Prasugrel
GP II_b/III_a antagonists
• Abciximab
• Eptifibatide
• Tirofiban

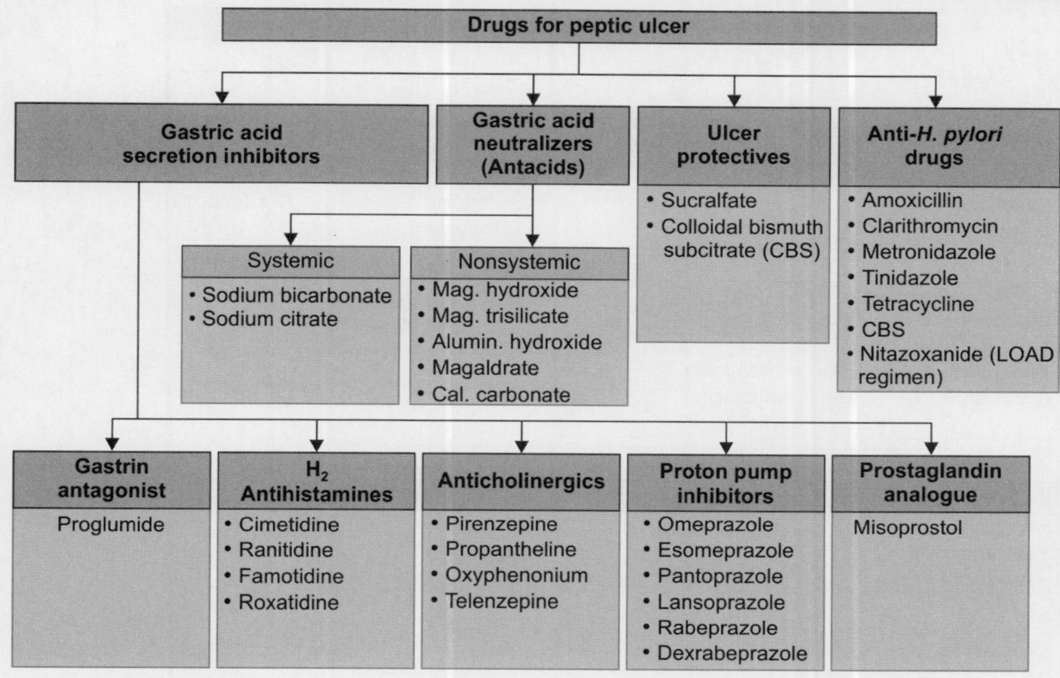
Drugs for peptic ulcer
Gastric acid secretion inhibitors
Gastric acid neutralizers (Antacids)
Ulcer protectives
• Sucralfate
• Colloidal bismuth subcitrate (CBS)
Anti-H. pylori drugs
• Amoxicillin
• Clarithromycin
• Metronidazole
• Tinidazole
• Tetracycline
• CBS
• Nitazoxanide (LOAD regimen)
Systemic
• Sodium bicarbonate
• Sodium citrate
Nonsystemic
• Mag. hydroxide
• Mag. trisilicate
• Alumin. hydroxide
• Magaldrate
• Cal. carbonate
Gastrin antagonist
Proglumide
H2 Antihistamines
• Cimetidine
• Ranitidine
• Famotidine
• Roxatidine
Anticholinergics
• Pirenzepine
• Propantheline
• Oxyphenonium
• Telenzepine
Proton pump inhibitors
• Omeprazole
• Esomeprazole
• Pantoprazole
• Lansoprazole
• Rabeprazole
• Dexrabeprazole
Prostaglandin analogue
Misoprostol

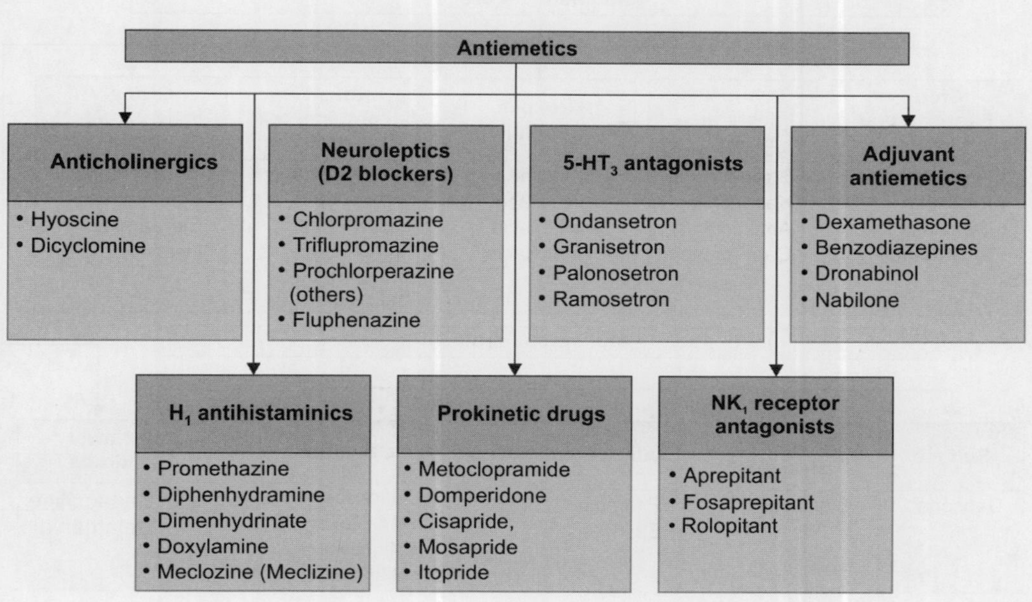
Antiemetics
Anticholinergics
• Hyoscine
• Dicyclomine
Neuroleptics (D2 blockers)
• Chlorpromazine
• Triflupromazine
• Prochlorperazine (others)
• Fluphenazine
5-HT3 antagonists
• Ondansetron
• Granisetron
• Palonosetron
• Ramosetron
Adjuvant antiemetics
• Dexamethasone
• Benzodiazepines
• Dronabinol
• Nabilone
H1 antihistaminics
• Promethazine
• Diphenhydramine
• Dimenhydrinate
• Doxylamine
• Meclozine (Meclizine)
Prokinetic drugs
• Metoclopramide
• Domperidone
• Cisapride,
• Mosapride
• Itopride
NK1 receptor antagonists
• Aprepitant
• Fosaprepitant
• Rolopitant

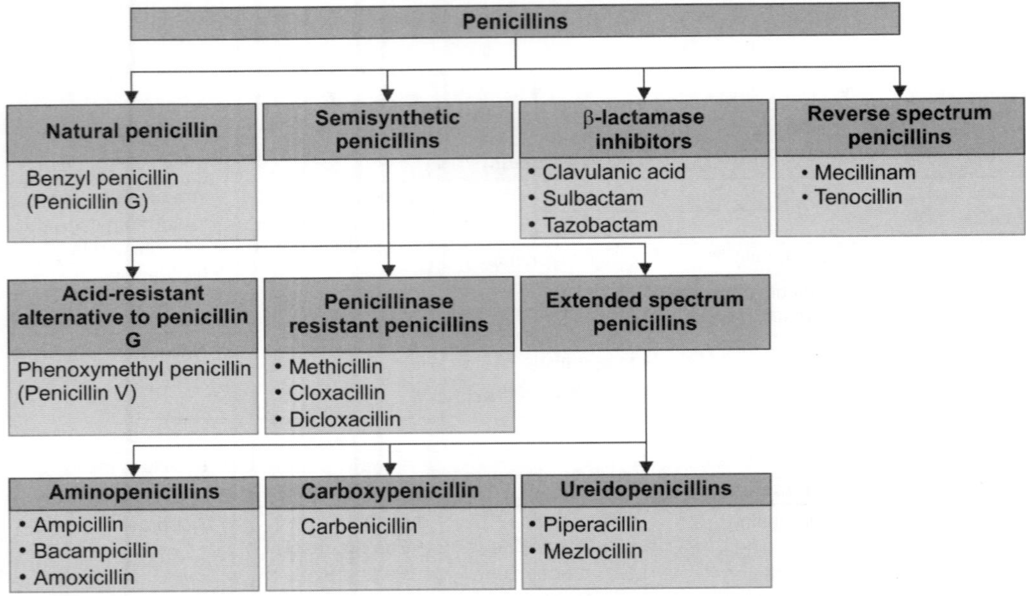
Penicillins
Natural penicillin
Benzyl penicillin (Penicillin G)
Semisynthetic penicillins
β-lactamase inhibitors
• Clavulanic acid
• Sulbactam
• Tazobactam
Reverse spectrum penicillins
• Mecillinam
• Tenocillin
Acid-resistant alternative to penicillin G
Phenoxymethyl penicillin (Penicillin V)
Penicillinase resistant penicillins
• Methicillin
• Cloxacillin
• Dicloxacillin
Extended spectrum penicillins
Aminopenicillins
• Ampicillin
• Bacampicillin
• Amoxicillin
Carboxypenicillin
Carbenicillin
Ureidopenicillins
• Piperacillin
• Mezlocillin

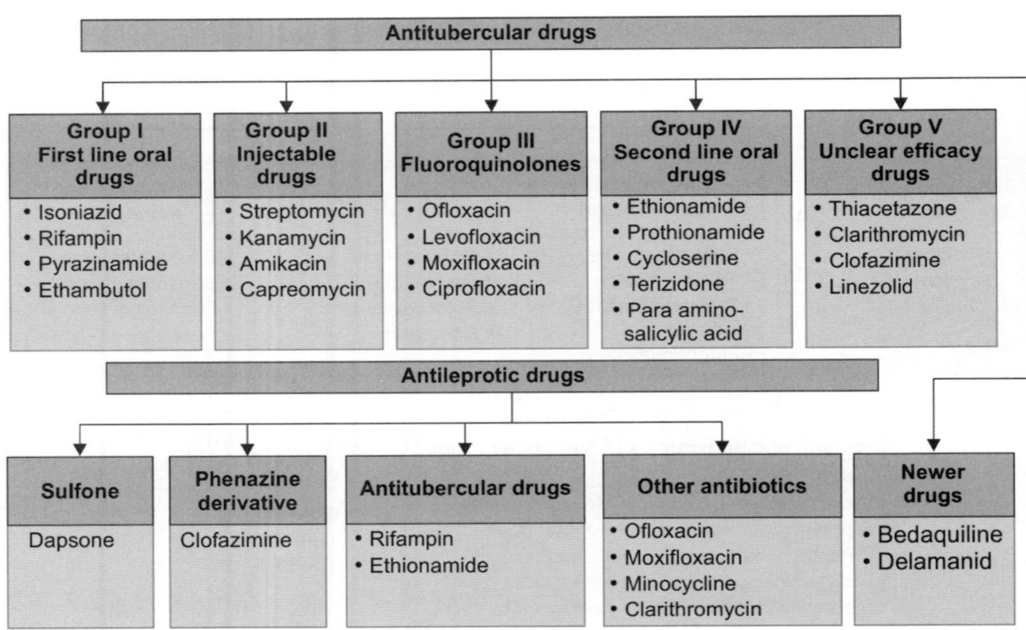
Antitubercular drugs
Group I First line oral drugs
• Isoniazid
• Rifampin
• Pyrazinamide
• Ethambutol
Group II Injectable drugs
• Streptomycin
• Kanamycin
• Amikacin
• Capreomycin
Group III Fluoroquinolones
• Ofloxacin
• Levofloxacin
• Moxifloxacin
• Ciprofloxacin
Group IV Second line oral drugs
• Ethionamide
• Prothionamide
• Cycloserine
• Terizidone
• Para amino-salicylic acid
Group V Unclear efficacy drugs
• Thiacetazone
• Clarithromycin
• Clofazimine
• Linezolid
Antileprotic drugs
Sulfone
Dapsone
Phenazine derivative
Clofazimine
Antitubercular drugs
• Rifampin
• Ethionamide
Other antibiotics
• Ofloxacin
• Moxifloxacin
• Minocycline
• Clarithromycin
Newer drugs
• Bedaquiline
• Delamanid

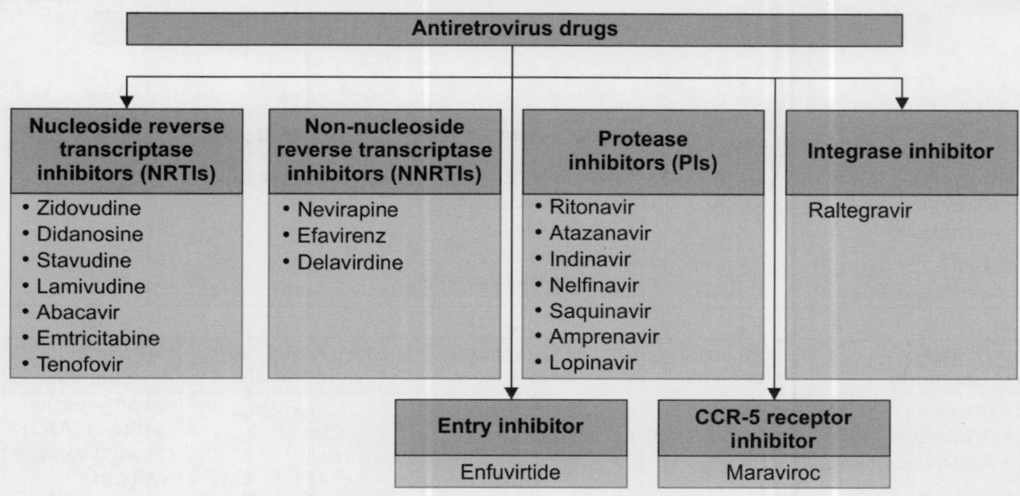
Antiretrovirus drugs
Nucleoside reverse transcriptase inhibitors (NRTIs)
• Zidovudine
• Didanosine
• Stavudine
• Lamivudine
• Abacavir
• Emtricitabine
• Tenofovir
Non-nucleoside reverse transcriptase inhibitors (NNRTIs)
• Nevirapine
• Efavirenz
• Delavirdine
Protease inhibitors (PIs)
• Ritonavir
• Atazanavir
• Indinavir
• Nelfinavir
• Saquinavir
• Amprenavir
• Lopinavir
Integrase inhibitor
Raltegravir
Entry inhibitor
Enfuvirtide
CCR-5 receptor inhibitor
Maraviroc

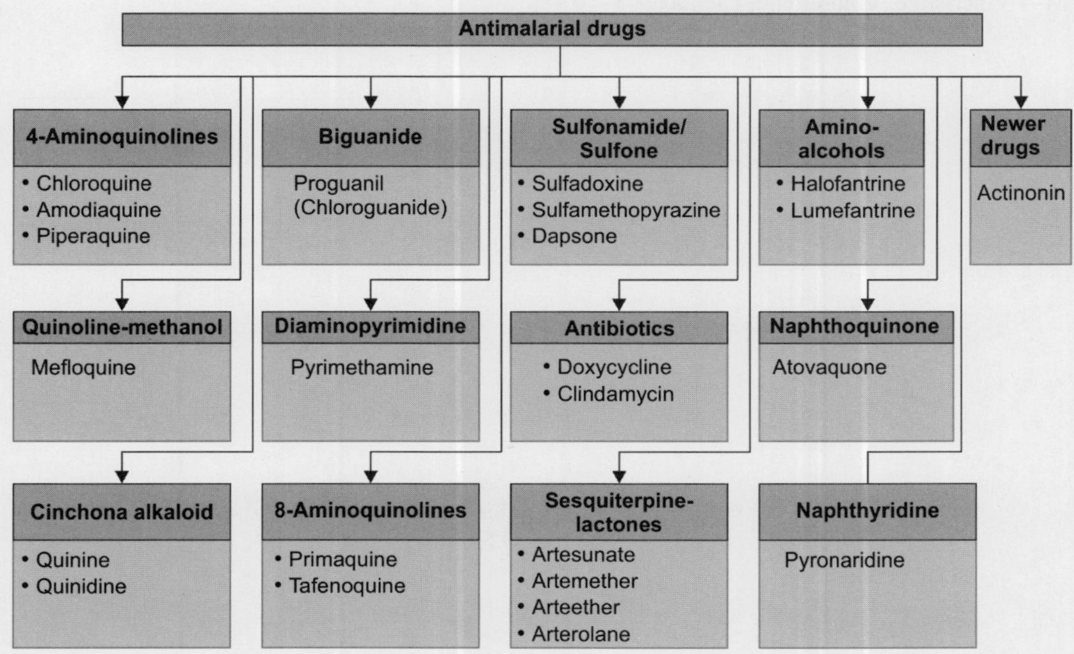
Antimalarial drugs
4-Aminoquinolines
• Chloroquine
• Amodiaquine
• Piperaquine
Biguanide
Proguanil (Chloroguanide)
Sulfonamide/ Sulfone
• Sulfadoxine
• Sulfamethopyrazine
• Dapsone
Amino-alcohols
• Halofantrine
• Lumefantrine
Newer drugs
Actinonin
Quinoline-methanol
Mefloquine
Diaminopyrimidine
Pyrimethamine
Antibiotics
• Doxycycline
• Clindamycin
Naphthoquinone
Atovaquone
Cinchona alkaloid
• Quinine
• Quinidine
8-Aminoquinolines
• Primaquine
• Tafenoquine
Sesquiterpine-lactones
• Artesunate
• Artemether
• Arteether
• Arterolane
Naphthyridine
Pyronaridine

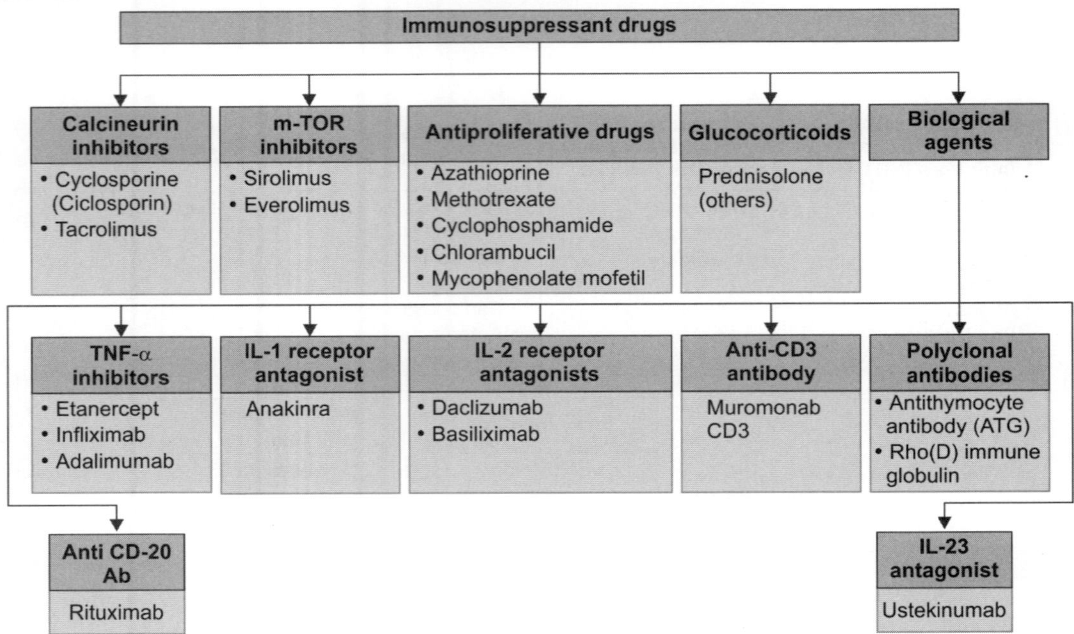

Classification of anticancer drugs according to cell cycle specificity:

G_1→ Vinblastine

S→ Mtx, cytanaleine, 6-TG, 5-FU, Doxorubicin, Mitomycine

G_2→ Bleomycin, Etoposide, Topotecan

M→ Vincristine, Vinorelbine, Paclitaxel

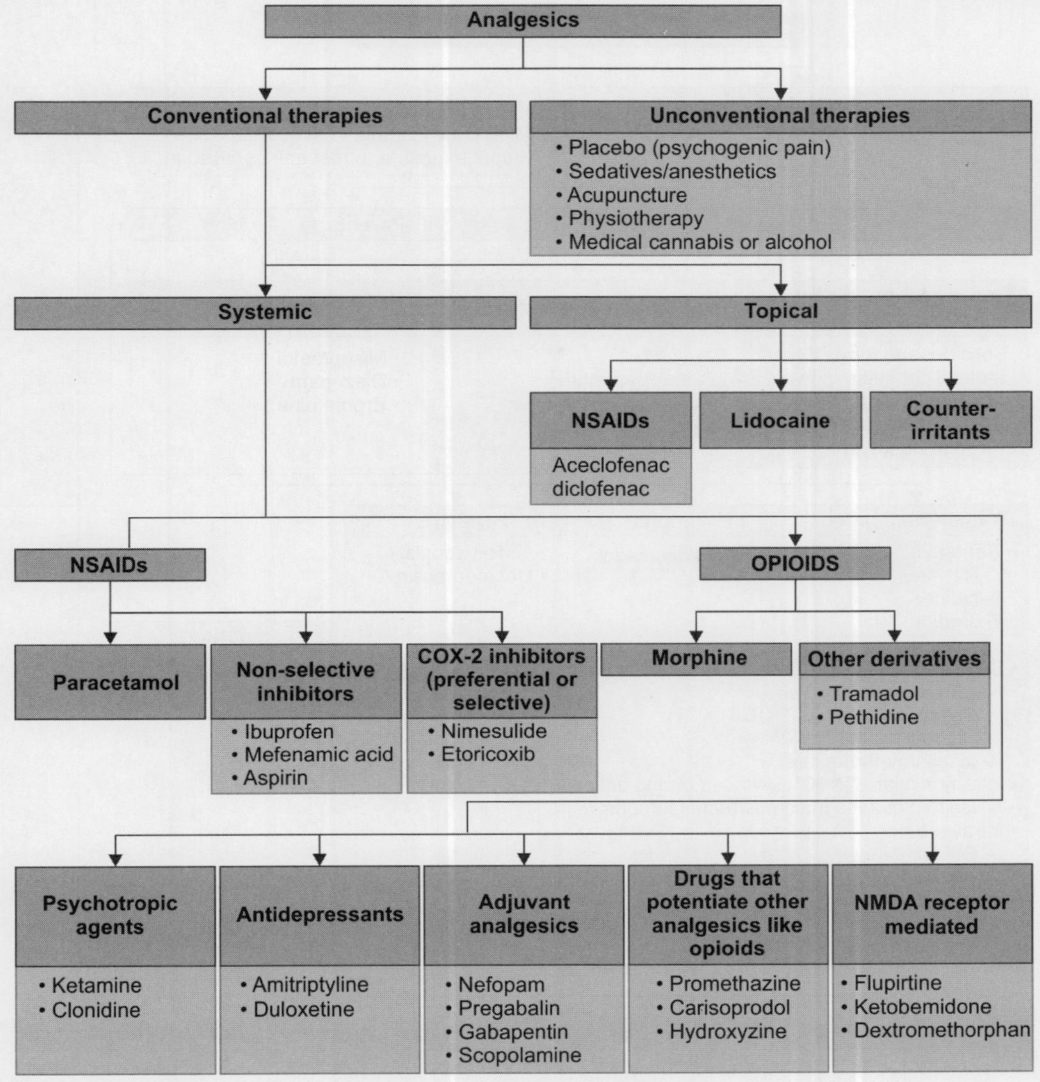
Analgesics
Conventional therapies
Unconventional therapies
• Placebo (psychogenic pain)
• Sedatives/anesthetics
• Acupuncture
• Physiotherapy
• Medical cannabis or alcohol
Systemic
Topical
NSAIDs
Aceclofenac
diclofenac
Lidocaine
Counter-irritants
NSAIDs
OPIOIDS
Paracetamol
Non-selective inhibitors
• Ibuprofen
• Mefenamic acid
• Aspirin
COX-2 inhibitors (preferential or selective)
• Nimesulide
• Etoricoxib
Morphine
Other derivatives
• Tramadol
• Pethidine
Psychotropic agents
• Ketamine
• Clonidine
Antidepressants
• Amitriptyline
• Duloxetine
Adjuvant analgesics
• Nefopam
• Pregabalin
• Gabapentin
• Scopolamine
Drugs that potentiate other analgesics like opioids
• Promethazine
• Carisoprodol
• Hydroxyzine
NMDA receptor mediated
• Flupirtine
• Ketobemidone
• Dextromethorphan

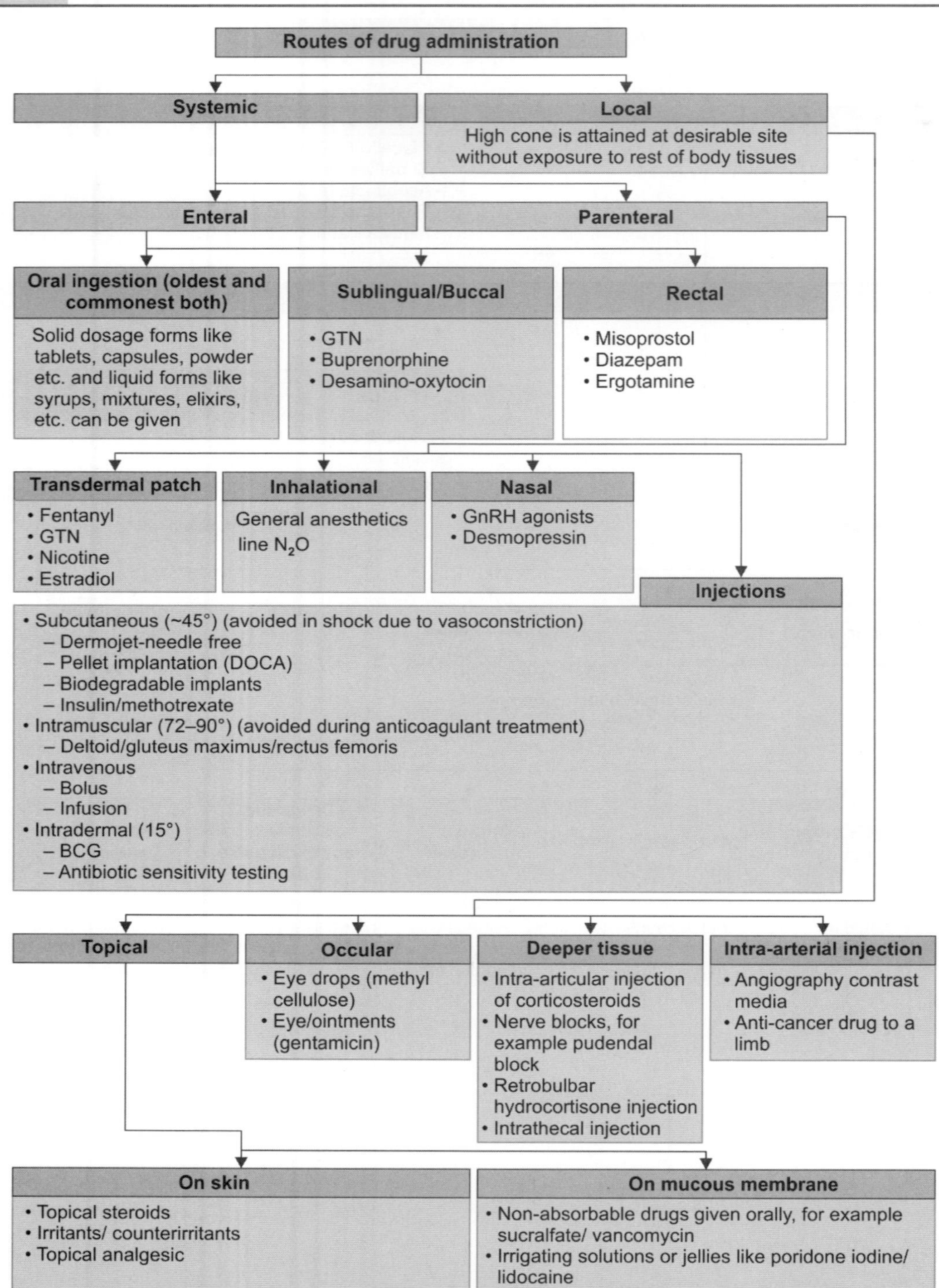
Routes of drug administration
Systemic
Local
High cone is attained at desirable site without exposure to rest of body tissues
Enteral
Parenteral
Oral ingestion (oldest and commonest both)
Solid dosage forms like tablets, capsules, powder etc. and liquid forms like syrups, mixtures, elixirs, etc. can be given
Sublingual/Buccal
• GTN
• Buprenorphine
• Desamino-oxytocin
Rectal
• Misoprostol
• Diazepam
• Ergotamine
Transdermal patch
• Fentanyl
• GTN
• Nicotine
• Estradiol
Inhalational
General anesthetics line N_2O
Nasal
• GnRH agonists
• Desmopressin
Injections
• Subcutaneous (~45°) (avoided in shock due to vasoconstriction)
– Dermojet-needle free
– Pellet implantation (DOCA)
– Biodegradable implants
– Insulin/methotrexate
• Intramuscular (72–90°) (avoided during anticoagulant treatment)
– Deltoid/gluteus maximus/rectus femoris
• Intravenous
– Bolus
– Infusion
• Intradermal (15°)
– BCG
– Antibiotic sensitivity testing
Topical
Occular
• Eye drops (methyl cellulose)
• Eye/ointments (gentamicin)
Deeper tissue
• Intra-articular injection of corticosteroids
• Nerve blocks, for example pudendal block
• Retrobulbar hydrocortisone injection
• Intrathecal injection
Intra-arterial injection
• Angiography contrast media
• Anti-cancer drug to a limb
On skin
• Topical steroids
• Irritants/ counterirritants
• Topical analgesic
On mucous membrane
• Non-absorbable drugs given orally, for example sucralfate/ vancomycin
• Irrigating solutions or jellies like poridone iodine/ lidocaine
• Inhalational cromolyn sodium

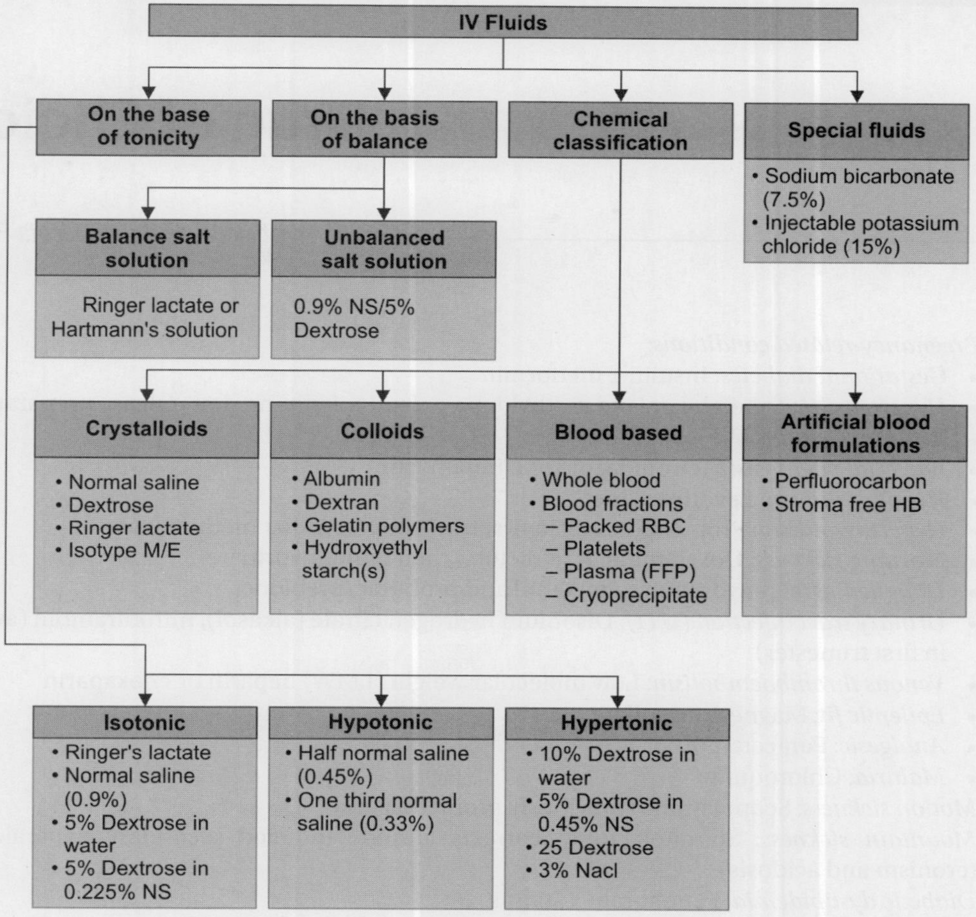
IV Fluids
On the base of tonicity
On the basis of balance
Chemical classification
Special fluids
• Sodium bicarbonate (7.5%)
• Injectable potassium chloride (15%)
Balance salt solution
Ringer lactate or Hartmann's solution
Unbalanced salt solution
0.9% NS/5% Dextrose
Crystalloids
• Normal saline
• Dextrose
• Ringer lactate
• Isotype M/E
Colloids
• Albumin
• Dextran
• Gelatin polymers
• Hydroxyethyl starch(s)
Blood based
• Whole blood
• Blood fractions
– Packed RBC
– Platelets
– Plasma (FFP)
– Cryoprecipitate
Artificial blood formulations
• Perfluorocarbon
• Stroma free HB
Isotonic
• Ringer's lactate
• Normal saline (0.9%)
• 5% Dextrose in water
• 5% Dextrose in 0.225% NS
Hypotonic
• Half normal saline (0.45%)
• One third normal saline (0.33%)
Hypertonic
• 10% Dextrose in water
• 5% Dextrose in 0.45% NS
• 25 Dextrose
• 3% Nacl

CHAPTER 3

Drug of Choice

Avishek Layek, Dyuti Deepta Rano

- *Pregnancy-related conditions*:
  - *Gestational diabetes*: Insulin ± metformin
  - *Hypertension*: Labetalol or/and methyldopa or/and nifedipine slow-release preparation
  - *Asthma*: Albuterol
  - *Bacterial vaginosis*: Metronidazole or clindamycin
  - *Hypothyroidism*: Levothyroxine
  - *Hyperthyroidism*: Propylthiouracil in first trimester, after that methimazole
  - *Morning sickness*: Doxylamine. If refractory, then dimenhydrinate
  - *Diarrhea*: Oral rehydration salts (ORS) and probiotic/prebiotics
  - *Urinary tract infection (UTI)*: Disodium hydrogen citrate (alkasol), nitrofurantoin (avoid in first trimester)
  - *Venous thromboembolism*: Low molecular weight (LMW) heparin or enoxaparin
  - *Epileptic fit*: Magnesium sulfate
  - *Analgesic*: Paracetamol
  - *Malaria*: Chloroquine
- *Motion sickness*: Scopolamine (previously promethazine)
- *Mountain sickness*: Spironolactone (corrects altitude induced secondary hyperaldosteronism and acidosis)
- *Diabetic dyslipidemia*: Fenofibrate ± statins
- *Infantile spasms*: Vigabatrin (valproate and clonazepam as adjuncts)
- *Absence seizures*: Valproate
- *Generalized tonic-clonic seizures (GTCS)*: Carbamazepine and phenytoin
- *Morphine withdrawal*: Methadone
- *Postoperative and radiation-induced vomiting*: Ondansetron
- *Smoking cessation*: Nicotine transdermal patch/varenicline/bupropion
- *Dysmenorrhea*: Ibuprofen [non-selective cyclooxygenase (COX)] and drotaverine
- *Simple headache*: Paracetamol
- *Paracetamol poisoning*: *N*-acetyl cysteine
- *Postoperative pain*: Tramadol
- *Carbamate poisoning*: Atropine
- *Atropine poisoning*: Physostigmine
- *Organophosphate (OP) poisoning*: Atropine (additionally oximes before aging occurs)
- *Cholera*: Doxycycline
- *Benzodiazepine (BZD) poisoning*: Flumazenil
- *Cheese reaction*: Phentolamine

- *Hypertension with benign prostatic hypertrophy (BHP)*: Prazosin
- *Malignant hyperthermia*: Dantrolene sodium
- *Methyl alcohol poisoning*: Fomepizole
- *Methicillin-resistant Staphylococcus aureus (MRSA)*: Vancomycin
- *Vancomycin-resistant Staphylococcus aureus (VRSA)*: Linezolid/streptogramins
- *Antipseudomonal*: Piperacillin + tazobactam
- *Postmenopausal osteoporosis*: Alendronate
- *Paroxysmal supraventricular tachycardia (PSVT)*: Adenosine
- *Cisplatin-induced vomiting*: Aprepitant
- *Bleeding esophageal varices*: Octreotide.

CHAPTER 4

Model Long Questions

Anusree Krishna Mandal

1. What is the treatment for acute thyrotoxicosis? Classify antithyroid drugs. Outline the preoperative drug therapy.

It is a systemic syndrome, which occurs as a result of excess production and release of thyroid hormones. It is an emergency requiring vigorous treatment.

General Measures

- Rehydration by intravenous (IV) infusion
- Anxiolytics
- External cooling
- Antibiotics.

Drug Treatment

- *Nonselective beta-blockers*: For example, Propranolol: 1–2 mg slow IV may be followed by oral therapy. They decrease the manifestations caused by sympathetic over activity. They also reduce peripheral conversion of T4 to T3.
- *Propylthiouracil*: 200–300 mg oral 6 hourly. It reduces both hormone synthesis and peripheral conversion from T4 to T3
- *Iopanoic acid/Ipodate*: 0.5–1 g OD oral. They inhibit both thyroid hormone release and peripheral conversion from T4 toT3
- *Corticosteroids*: Hydrocortisone 100 mg IV 8 hourly followed by oral prednisolone. These help tide over crisis, covers adrenal insufficiency and inhibit peripheral conversion of T4 to T3
- *Diltiazem*: 60–120 mg BD oral may be added if beta blockers are not sufficient to control tachycardia or are contraindicated.

Classification

It is given in Chapter 2 for surgery,

Preoperative Drug Treatment

- Thioamides at least for 2–3 weeks
- Iodide for 10 days
- If indicated, propranolol orally
- A euthyroid state is produced and operative mortality is reduced.

During the therapy, thioamide is administered before iodide because prior administration of iodide may prevent thioamide induced activation of thyroid peroxidases.

2. Classify antiepileptic drugs. What is the mechanism of action of phenytoin? What are its side effects?

The classification of antiepileptic drugs is given in Chapter 2.

Mechanism of Action of Phenytoin

- At therapeutic concentrations:

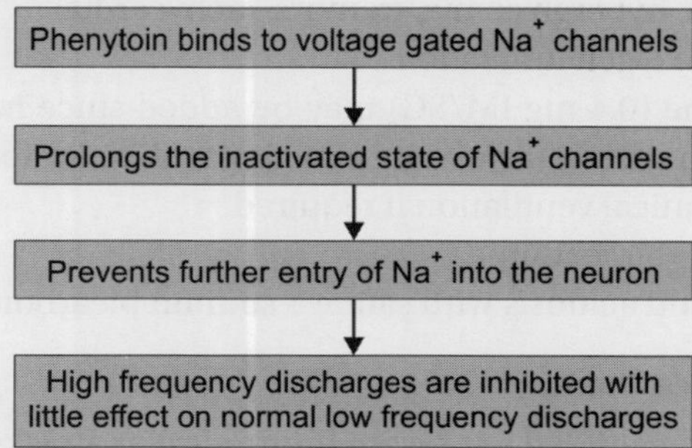

- *At higher toxic concentrations, other effects are*:
  - Reduction in calcium influx and inhibition of glutamate and facilitation of gamma-aminobutyric acid (GABA) responses
  - Phenytoin does not interfere with kindling.

Side Effects

- At therapeutic dose (10–20 μg/mL): [Mnemonics—H(4)OT MALIKA]
  - Hirsutism
  - Hyperplasia of gums
  - Hypersensitivity
  - Hyperglycemia
  - Osteomalacia
  - Teratogenic—fetal hydantoin syndrome
  - Megaloblastic anemia
- At toxic doses (>20 μg/mL): (Mnemonics—BCDEFH)
  Behavioral disturbances, Cerebellar signs, Drowsiness, Epigastric pain, Fall in BP, Hallucinations.

3. Outline the management of status asthmaticus. What are drugs to be used in maintenance therapy to reduce frequency of attacks? Classify drugs used in bronchial asthma.

Management of Status Asthmaticus

- Hydrocortisone hemisuccinate 100 mg IV stat, followed by 100–200 mg 4–8 hourly infusion.
  Mechanism of action: Pure anti-inflammatory action—induction of annexins, negative regulation of COX-2 and genes for cytokines, decreased production of acute phase reactants and decreased expression of transcription factors.
  Thus they act by reducing bronchial hyperactivity, mucosal edema and by suppressing inflammation.

- Nebulized salbutamol (2.5–5 mg) + ipratropium bromide (0.5 mg) intermittent inhalations driven by O_2.
  Mechanism of action: Beta-2 agonist → Increase in cAMP in bronchial smooth muscles → Relaxation
  Also, increased cAMP in mast cells → Decreased mediators release.

Side effects: Hypokalemia, hyperglycemia, tremors, tachycardia

- High flow humidified oxygen inhalation
- Salbutamol/terbutaline (0.4 mg IM/SC) may be added since inhaled drug may not reach smaller bronchi due to severe narrowing/plugging with secretions.
- Intubation and mechanical ventilation if required.
- Antibiotics for any chest infection
- Correct dehydration and acidosis with saline + sodium bicarbonate/lactate infusion.

Drug Used in Maintenance Therapy

The drugs which can be prescribed to prevent future similar attacks or for maintenance are:

- Formoterol
- Salmeterol
- Bambuterol
- Theophylline
- Sodium cromoglicate (SCG).

Classification of drugs: It is given in Chapter 2.

GINA (GLOBAL STRATEGY FOR ASTHMA MANAGEMENT AND PREVENTION 2016 UPDATE)

Definition of Asthma

Asthma is a heterogeneous disease, usually characterized by chronic airway inflammation. It is defined by the history of respiratory symptoms such as wheeze, shortness of breath, chest tightness and cough that vary over time and in intensity, together with variable expiratory airflow limitation.

Definition of Asthma Exacerbations

Exacerbations of asthma are episodes characterized by a progressive increase in symptoms of shortness of breath, cough, wheezing or chest tightness and progressive decrease in lung function, i.e. they represent a change from the patient's usual status that is sufficient to require a change in treatment. Exacerbations may occur in patients with a pre-existing diagnosis of asthma or, occasionally, as the first presentation of asthma. Exacerbations usually occur in response to exposure to an external agent (e.g. viral upper respiratory tract infection, pollen or pollution) and/or poor adherence with controller medication; however, a subset of patients present more acutely and without exposure to known risk factors. Severe exacerbations can occur in patients with mild or well-controlled asthma.

Management of Acute Attack (Status Asthmaticus)

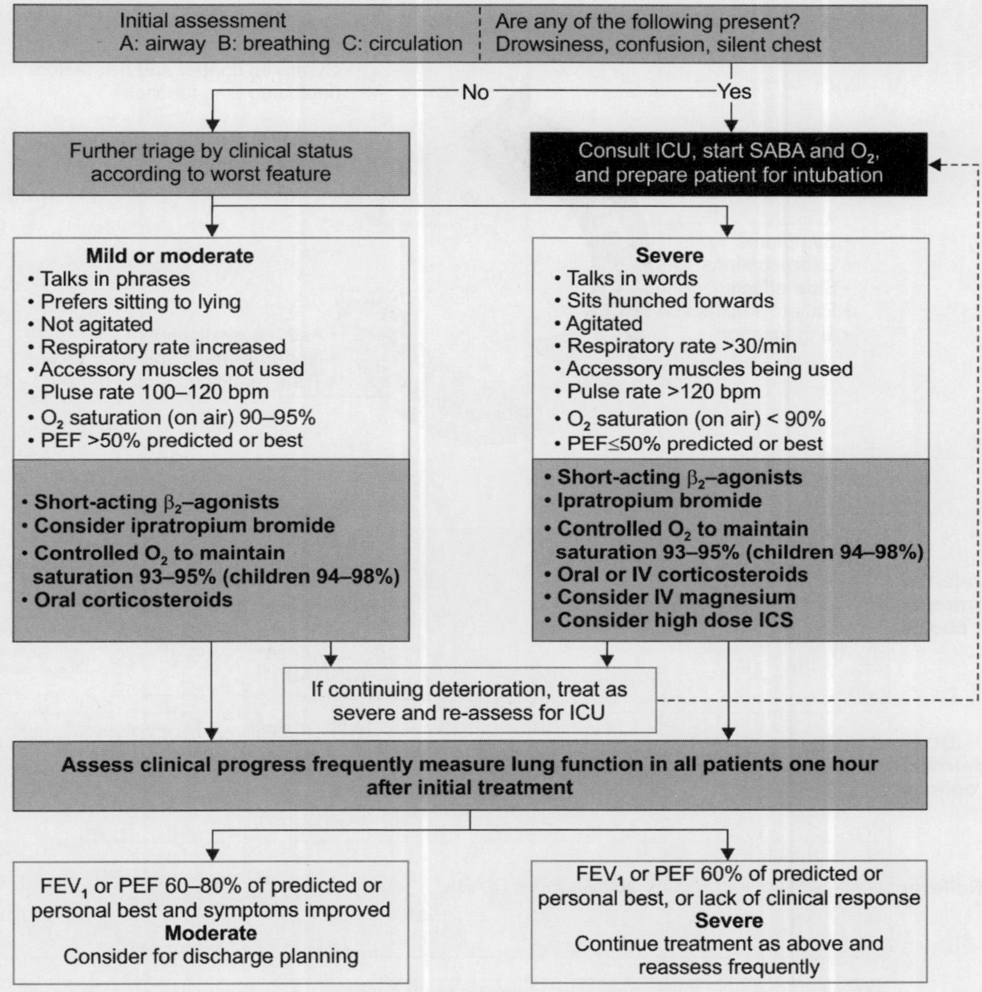

Abbreviations: ICS, inhaled corticosteroids; ICU, intensive care unit; IV, intravenous; O_2, oxygen; PEF, peak expiratory flow FEV_1, forced expiratory volume in 1 second

Management of Chronic Asthma (Step-up and Down Approach)

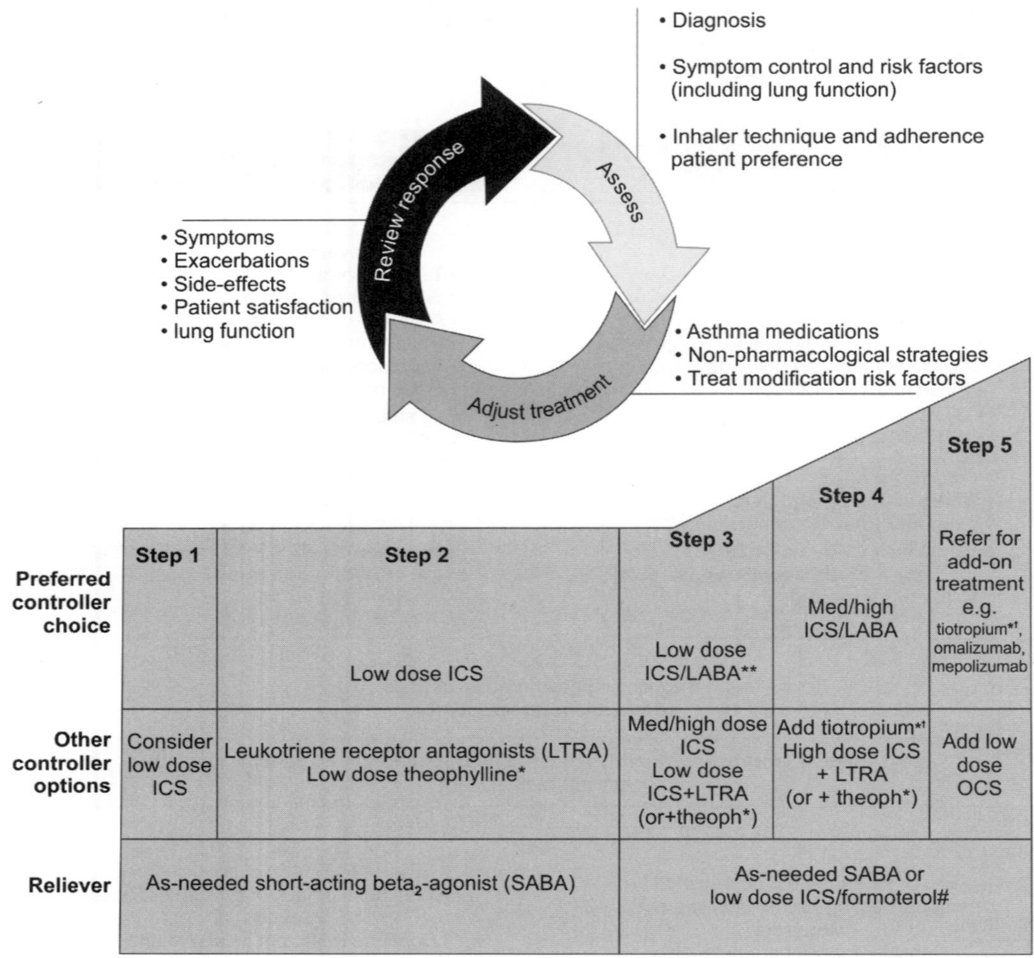

	Step 1	Step 2	Step 3	Step 4	Step 5
Preferred controller choice		Low dose ICS	Low dose ICS/LABA**	Med/high ICS/LABA	Refer for add-on treatment e.g. tiotropium*†, omalizumab, mepolizumab
Other controller options	Consider low dose ICS	Leukotriene receptor antagonists (LTRA) Low dose theophylline*	Med/high dose ICS Low dose ICS+LTRA (or+theoph*)	Add tiotropium*† High dose ICS + LTRA (or + theoph*)	Add low dose OCS
Reliever	As-needed short-acting beta$_2$-agonist (SABA)		As-needed SABA or low dose ICS/formoterol#		

Remember to...

- Provide guided self-management education (self-monitoring + written action plan + regular review)
- Treat modifiable risk factors and comorbidities, e.g. smoking, obesity, anxiety
- Advise about non-pharmacological therapies and strategies, e.g. physical activity, weight loss, avoidance of sensitizers where appropriate
- Consider stepping up if ...uncontrolled symptoms, exacerbations or risks, but check diagnosis, inhaler techniques and adherence first
- Consider stepping down if ...symptoms controlled for 3 months + low risk for exacerbations
- Ceasing ICS is not advised

Abbreviations: ICS, inhaled corticosteroids; LABA, long-acting beta2-agonist; med, medium dose; OCS, oral corticosteroids

4. Outline the management of congestive cardiac failure (CCF). Classify drugs used in CCF. What are the cardiac side effects of digitalis therapy? Name the drugs causing torsades de pointes.

Management of Congestive Cardiac Failure

- Rest is advised
- Moderate salt restriction (2–3 g/day)
- Tablet frusemide (20–80 mg/day) to be added and tablet spironolactone (25 mg/day)
- *Tablet enalapril*: Start with a low dose of 2.5 mg daily after stopping diuretic for 1–2 days. If there is no hypotension, dose can be gradually increased to 40 mg/day depending on the response.
- Cause of heart failure to be investigated and treated if possible.
- Serum potassium to be monitored at regular intervals and supplementation to be given accordingly.

Classification of drugs used in congestive cardiac failure is given in Chapter 2.

Possible Cardiac Toxic Effects of Digitalis Therapy

- *Vagomimetic action*: Bradycardia, AV block
- *Almost every type of arrhythmia*: Tachyarrhythmia, supraventricular arrhythmia, ventricular arrhythmia, AV block
- *Early indications of toxicity*: GI symptoms (nausea, vomiting).

Drugs causing Torsades de Pointes

The drugs causing torsades de pointes are given in Table 4.1.

Table 4.1: Drugs that prolong Q-T interval (have potential to precipitate torsades de pointes)

Antiarrhythmics	Quinidine, procainamide, disopyramide, propafenone, amiodarone
Antimalarials	Quinine, mefloquine, artemisinin, halofantrine
Antibacterials	Sparfloxacin, moxifloxacin
Antihistaminics	Terfenadine, astemizole, ebastine
Antidepressants	Amitriptyline and other tricyclics
Antipsychotics	Thioridazine, pimozide, aripiprazole, ziprasidone
Prokinetic	Cisapride

5. Outline the signs, symptoms and management of datura poisoning. Classify cholinomimetic drugs. Name some uses of cholinergic agonists.

Datura Poisoning

Active ingredient: Atropine and hyoscine.

Signs and Symptoms

- Rapid and weak pulse
- Dry mouth

- Dilatation of pupil
- Blurred vision
- Hot, dry, and scarlet skin
- Excitement, delirium, and hallucinations.

Hot as hare, red as a beet, dry as a bone, blind as a bat, and mad as a hen/hatter.

Pharmacological Basis of Treatment

Main Treatment

Physostigmine salicylate: 1–4 mg in adult and 0.5 mg in children as slow IV.

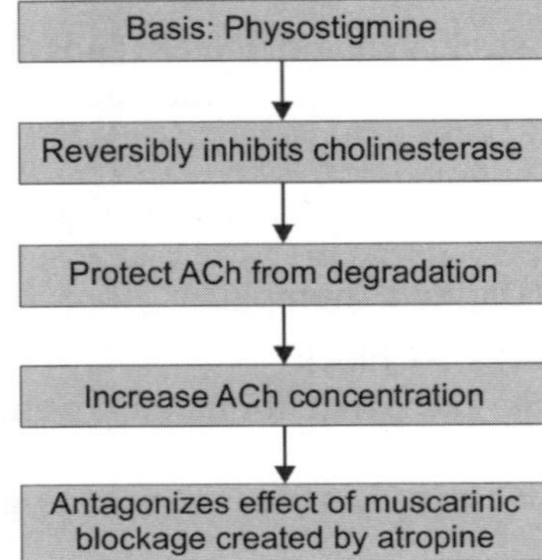

Physostigmine can cross blood-brain barrier and acts both centrally and peripherally.
Other treatment options are:

- *Diazepam*: To treat convulsions and excitement
- *Lignocaine*: For ventricular arrhythmia
- *Classification* of cholinomimetic drugs is given in Chapter 2.

Uses of Cholinergic Agonists

- Pilocarpine is used in both types of glaucoma
- *Bethanechol:* Postoperative/partum, nonobstructive urinary retention; congenital megacolon; gastroesophageal reflux disease (GERD) (rarely used now)
- *Methacoline:* Termination of paroxysmal supraventricular tachycardia (PSVT) (rarely used now)
- ACh is not used because of its evanescent and nonselective action.

6. Classify drugs used in glaucoma. Outline the treatment of acute attack of angle-closure glaucoma. What are the advantages of topical beta-blockers over miotics?

The classification of drugs used in glaucoma is given in Chapter 2. The management of acute attack has been described in Chapter 9.

Advantages of Topical Beta-blockers Over Miotics

- *No change in pupil size*: No diminution of vision in dim light and in patients with cataract
- No induced myopia which is especially troublesome in young patients
- No headache/brow pain due to persistent spasm of iris and ciliary muscles

- No fluctuations in intra-occular tension (IOT) as occur with pilocarpine drops
- Convenient twice/once daily application sufficient.

7. Enumerate antihypertensive drugs. Outline the management of hypertensive emergency. What are the side effects of angiotensin-converting-enzyme inhibitor (ACEI)?

The classification of antihypertensive drugs is given in Chapter 2 and the management of hypertensive emergency is described in Chapter 9.

Side effects of angiotensin-converting-enzyme inhibitor (ACEI)

- *Hypotension:* Initial sharp fall in BP
- Hyperkalemia
- Persistent codeine resistant cough
- Rashes and utricaria
- Angioedema
- Dysgeusia
- Fetopathic
- Headache, dizziness, nausea and bowel upset
- Granulocytopenia and proteinuria
- *Acute renal failure:* In patients with bilateral renal artery stenosis (absolute contraindication).

8. Classify the drugs used in angina pectoris. Outline the mechanism of action of nitrates. Outline the management of stable angina.

The classification of drugs used in angina pectoris is given in Chapter 2. The mechanism of action of nitrates is described in Chapter 6 and management of stable angina is described in Chapter 9.

9. Mention different insulin preparations. How will you manage a case of hypoglycemic coma? What are the side effects and indications for insulin therapy?

The different insulin preparations are given in Chapter 2 and the management of hypoglycemic coma is described in Chapter 9.

Indications of Insulin Therapy

- Type 1 diabetes mellitus (DM)
- Diabetic ketoacidosis
- Hyperglycemic hyperosmolar non-ketotic coma
- Uncontrolled type 2 DM previously on oral hypoglycemic agents (OHA)
- Gestational DM
- Controlled type 2 DM female who has now become pregnant
- Any period of crisis, such as surgery, trauma, stress, etc., which temporarily increases insulin demand in body in a type 2 DM patient on OHA.

Side Effects

- Hypoglycemia
- Local reactions

- Lipodystrophy (atrophy due to reaction and hypertrophy due to insulin growth factor mediated growth)
- Allergy
- Edema
- Weight gain.

10. Classify corticosteroids. What are the side effects and contraindications of glucocorticoid therapy? How to minimize HPA axis suppression? Name a glucocorticoid antagonist.

The classification of corticosteroids is given in Chapter 2.

Side Effects

- Cushing's habitus
- Fragile skin, purple striae, easy bruising, telengiectasia
- Hirsutism
- Hyperglycemia and DM precipitation
- Muscular weakness primarily proximal
- Increased susceptibility to infections
- Delayed wound healing
- Peptic ulceration
- Osteoporosis and spontaneous fractures
- Posterior subcapsular cataract
- Glaucoma
- Growth retardation
- Fetal abnormalities
- Psychiatric disturbances and decreased seizure threshold
- Hypothalamic-pituitary-adrenal (HPA) axis suppression.

Contraindications

The following diseases are aggravated by corticosteroids. Since corticosteroids may have to be used as a lifesaving measure, all of these are relative contraindications in the presence of which these drugs are to be employed only under compelling circumstances and with due precautions.

- Peptic ulcer
- Diabetes mellitus
- Hypertension
- Viral and fungal infections
- Tuberculosis and other infections
- Osteoporosis
- Herpes simplex keratitis
- Psychosis
- Epilepsy
- CHF
- Renal failure.

Steps to Minimize Hypothalamic Pituitary Adrenal Axis Suppression

Measures that minimize HPA axis suppression are:

- Use shorter-acting steroids (hydrocortisone prednisolone) at the lowest possible dose
- Use steroids for the shortest period of time possible
- Give, the entire daily dose at one time in the morning
- Switch to alternate-day therapy if possible.

  It has been found that moderate dose of a short-acting steroid (e.g. prednisolone) given at 48 hours interval did not cause HPA suppression, whereas the same total amount given in four divided 12 hourly doses produced marked HPA suppression. Alternate-day therapy also resulted in less immunological suppression—lower risk of infection. The longer-acting steroids (dexamethasone, etc.) are not suitable for alternate-day therapy. Only problem with alternate-day therapy is that many steroid dependent patients are incapacitated on the *off day*.
- If appropriate, use local (dermal, inhaled, ocular, nasal, rectal, intrasynovial) preparations of a steroid with poor systemic availability (beclomethasone, triamcinolone acetonide fluticasone, etc.)

Glucocorticoid receptor antagonist: Mifepristone.

CHAPTER 5

Short Notes

Anusree Krishna Mandal

GENERAL PHARMACOLOGY

Essential Drugs

- *WHO definition:* Those drugs, which satisfy the priority healthcare needs of the population. They are selected with due regard to public health relevance, evidence on efficacy and safety and comparative cost effectiveness.
- They are intended to be available within the context of functioning health systems at all times and in adequate amounts in appropriate dosage forms, with assured quality and adequate information and a price, so that the individual and the community can afford.
- WHO brought out its first *Model List of Essential Drugs* in 1977 which could be adopted after suitable modifications according to local needs.
- In India, its current edition is *18th National List of Essential Medicines*. It was revised in 2013 and contains 406 drugs.
- A few criteria given by WHO to guide the selection of essential medicines are:
  - Adequate data on efficacy and safety should be available.
  - Available in a form in which quality can be assured.
  - Choice depends on prevalent diseases.
  - Cost-benefit ratio
  - Local facilities
  - Single compounds preferred over fixed dose combinations.
  - Rationally developed treatment guidelines should also be considered.
- Example of essential drugs are amoxicillin, bisoprolol, carbamazepine, colchicine, dapsone, etc.

Orphan Drugs

- *Definition*: Drugs or biological products for diagnosis/treatment/prevention of a rare disease or condition or a more common disease (endemic only in resource poor countries) for which there is no reasonable expectation that the cost of developing and marketing it will be recovered from the sales of that drug.
- The disease itself is sometimes known as orphan disease.
- *Examples*: Sodium nitrite, fomepizole, miltefosine, somatropine, etc.
- They are commercially difficult to obtain.
- Governments in developed countries offer tax benefits and incentives to companies for developing and marketing orphan drugs, e.g. Orphan Drug Act in USA.

Physical Redistribution of Drugs

- Highly lipid soluble drugs get initially distributed to organs with high blood flow, i.e. brain, heart, kidney, etc. Later, less vascular but more bulky tissues (muscles, fat) take up the drug leading to fall in plasma concentration, and the drug is withdrawn from the highly perfused sites. This is known as redistribution.
- If the site of action of the drugs was in one of the highly perfused organs, redistribution results in termination of drug action.
- Greater the lipid solubility, faster is its redistribution.
- *Examples*: (a) Thiopentone sodium (IV)—Redistribution $t_{1/2}$ = 3 minutes (b) Oral diazepam or nitrazepam.

However, the same drug is is given repeatedly over long periods, the low perfusion high capacity sites get filled up and drug becomes longer acting.

Therapeutic Index or Safety Margin

- *Definition*: It is a measure of the safety of the drug. Graphically, it is the gap between the therapeutic effect DRC and the adverse effect DRC.
- *Mathematically,*

$$TI = LD50/ED50$$

  - *ED50 (median effective dose)*: Dose that will produce half the maximum (50%) response. More the ED50, lower is the potency.
  - *MD50 (median lethal dose)*: Dose that will results in the death of 50% of the recipients. More the MD50, safer is the drug.
  - *Drugs having low TI*: Aminoglycoside, TCA, antiarrhythmics, digoxin, lithium, etc. These drugs require TDP or therapeutic dose monitoring.
  - Drugs having greater TI—Benzodiazepines.
  - Drugs having narrow TI have steep DRC slope (e.g. barbiturates) and those having broader TI have less steep DRC curves (e.g. BZPs)
- *Uses*: It gives an idea about the potential effectiveness and safety of the drug in human beings.
- Higher the TI, safer is the drug and vice versa.
- Clinically, I = Maximum tolerated dose/maximum curative dose.

Enzyme Induction

- *Introduction*: Enzyme induction refers to increase in the synthesis of microsomal enzyme protein due to interaction with another substance leading to increased metabolism of inducing drug itself and /or other drugs.
- *Examples*: Different inducers are relatively selective for certain cytochrome p-450 families:
  - Anticonvulsants, rifampicin induce CYP3A isoenzymes.
  - Phenobarbitone induce CYP2B1 and rifampicin also induce CYP2D6.
  - Isoniazid and chronic alcoholism induce CYP2E1.
- Induction involves microsomal enzymes in liver as well as other organs and increases rate of metabolism by 2–4-fold. Induction takes 4–14 days to reach its peak and is maintained till the inducing agent is given. Thereafter, the enzymes return to their original value over 1–3 weeks.

Receptor Antagonism

- *Introduction*: In this type of antagonism, one drug (antagonist) blocks the receptor action of the other (agonist). Receptor antagonists are relatively selective.
- *Types*:
  - *Competitive antagonism*: Antagonist which is chemically similar to the agonist competes with it and binds to the same site as agonist.
    - Binding is reversible and depends on the relative concentrations of antagonist and agonist.
    - *Example*: Ach and atropine, morphine and naloxone.
  - *Noncompetitive antagonism*: The antagonist which is chemically unrelated to the agonist, binds to a different allosteric site altering the receptor in such a way that it is unable to combine with the agonist.
    - Reversal of the antagonism can be done by increasing agent concentration.
    - *Example*: Diazepam and bicuculline.
  - *Irreversible or nonequilibrium antagonism*: Antagonist binds to the receptor with strong bonds or dissociate from it slowly so that agonist molecules are unable to reduce receptor occupancy of antagonist molecules.
    - Refer to Figure 4.19; p.59; KDT
- *Consequences*: The consequences are as follows:
  - Decreased intensity and/or duration of action of drugs, e.g. failure of contraception with OCPs.
  - Increase intensity of action of drugs that are activated by metabolism, e.g. acute paracetamol toxicity.
  - Tolerance
  - Precipitation of acute intermittent porphyria by depression of gamma aminolevulinic synthetase.
- *Possible uses*: Following are the possible uses:
  - Congenital nonhemolytic jaundice
  - Cushing's syndrome
  - Chronic poisoning
  - Liver disease.

Partial Agonist and Inverse Agonist

- *Partial agonist*: It activates the receptor submaximally. It will produce the similar effect in the absence of agonist but it will decrease the effect of a pure agonist.
  - *Example*: Pindolol has partial agonistic activity at beta-1 receptors. It produces antagonistic effect in presence of agonists like adrenaline and nor-adrenaline, i.e. decreases heart rate but even in high doses it does not produce severe bradycardia
  - *Intrinsic activity*: Between 0 and +1
- *Inverse agonist*: These drugs bind to the receptor and produce opposite effect.
  - *Example*: Beta carboline at benzodiazepine receptor
  - *Intrinsic activity*: Negative.

Drug Synergism

- *Etymology*: Greek— *Syn*: together; *Ergon*: work
- *Definition*: When the action of one drug is facilitated or increased by the other, they are said to be synergistic.

- *Types*: It can be of two types:
  1. *Additive*: The effect of the two drugs is in the same direction and simply adds up.
     - Effect of drugs A + B = Effect of drug A + Effect of drug B
     - *Examples*:
       - Aspirin + Paracetamol— Analgesic/antipyretic
       - Amlodipine + Atenolol—Antihypertensive
       - Ephedrine + Theophylline—Bronchodilator
       - Glibenclamide + Metformin—Hypoglycemic
  2. *Supraadditive (potentiation): The effect of combination is greater than the individual effects of the components.*
     - Effect of drug A+B > Effect of drug A+Effect of drug N
     - This is the case when one component given alone produces no effect but enhances the effect of the other.

Pharmacovigilance

- *WHO definition* (2002): Science and activities relating to the detection, assessment, understanding and prevention of adverse effects or any other drug related problem.
- *Purpose*: Its main purpose is to reduce risk of drug related harm to the patient.
- *Activities*: The activities involved are:
  - Post-marketing surveillance and other methods of ADR monitoring. Voluntary reporting depends on the initiative and willingness of the health professionals.
  - Dissemination of ADR data through 'drug alerts,' 'medical letters,' etc.
  - Changes in labeling of medicines indicating restrictions.
- *Pharmacovigilance centers*: They have been put up in many countries, e.g India (Central Drugs Standard Control Organization—CDSCO)
- *Casuality assessment*: It is assessed on the basis of:
  - Temporal relationship
  - Previous knowledge
  - Dechallenge
  - Rechallenge.

  Assessed on the basis of above criteria, causality has been graded as:
  - Definite
  - Probable
  - Possible
  - Doubtful.

First-pass Metabolism

- *Definition*: First-pass metabolism (FPM) refers to metabolism of a drug during its passage from the site of absorption into the systemic circulation. It is also called presystemic metabolism.
- All orally administered drugs are exposed to drug metabolizing enzymes in the intestinal wall and liver.
- Presystemic metabolism can also occur in the skin and in lungs.

- *Features of drugs with high FPM are*:
  - Oral dose is considerably higher than sublingual or parenteral dose
  - There is marked individual variation in the oral dose due to difference in the extent of FPM
  - Oral bioavailability of a drug is increased if another drug competing with its FPM is given concurrently
  - Liver diseases leads to increase in oral bioavailability
- *Examples*:
  - *Low FPM*: Phenobarbitone, phenylbutazone, tolbutamide, theophylline.
  - *Intermediate FPM*: aspirin, chlorpromazine, metoprolol.
  - *High FPM*: Hydrocortisone, verapamil, salbutamol, morphine, nitroglycerin.

Plasma Protein Binding of Drugs

- *Description:*
  - Acidic drugs bind with albumin but basic drugs bind with alpha 1 acid glycoprotein. In addition, there are some special globulins (transferrin, ceruloplasmin, TBG).
  - Protein-bound drugs are pharmacologically inactive, nondiffusible, nonmetabolized and non-excreted.
  - Protein bindings act as a temporary storage of drugs.
  - Drugs bind to plasma protein reversibly. This is a dynamic equilibrium between the free and bound form of the drugs.
- When plasma concentration of the free drug falls, the equilibrium is maintained by immediate release of the drugs from protein binding sites.
- *Examples*:
  - *High plasma protein bound*: Diazepam, propranolol, phenytoin, doxycycline, tolbutamide.
  - *Low plasma protein bound*: Lithium, ethosuximide.
- *Clinical significance*:
  - Higher the protein binding, longer the duration of action.
  - Highly protein-bound drugs are largely restricted to vascular apartment and have low Vd.
  - In hypoproteinemia, the dose of the highly protein-bound drugs should be properly adjusted.
  - When two drugs have high affinity for the same binding sites, then on simultaneous administration, clinically important drugs interactions may occur.
  - Highly protein-bound drugs are less effective in acute condition.

Plasma Half-life

- *Definition*: The plasma half-life of a drug is the time taken for its plasma concentration to be reduced to half of its original value.
- It is denoted by $t_{1/2}$.
- Mathematically,

$$t_{1/2} = \ln/k, \text{ where, } k = \text{elimination rate constant of the drug.}$$

$$\text{Or } t_{1/2} = 0.693 \times Vd/CL$$

- As such, $t_{1/2}$ is a derived parameter from two variables Vd and Cl, both of which may change independently. Thus, it is not an exact index of drug elimination.
- Complete drug elimination occurs in 4–5 half-lives.

- For drugs eliminated by:
  - *First-order kinetics*: $t_{1/2}$ remains constant.
  - *Zero-order kinetics*: $t_{1/2}$ increases with dose.
- *Examples*:
  - *Aspirin*: 4 hours
  - *Doxycycline*: 20 hours
  - *Digoxin*: 40 hours.

Loading Dose

- *Definition*: This is a single or few quickly repeated doses given in the beginning to attain target concentration rapidly.
- Mathematically,

$$\text{Loading dose} = Cp \times Vd/F,$$

where

Cp = target plasma concentration, Vd = volume of distribution and F = bioavailability

  - Thus, LD is governed only by Vd and not CL or $t_{1/2}$
  - LD is generally followed by maintenance dose.
  - Such two-phase dosing provides rapid therapeutic effect with long-term safety.
- Drugs given like that are digoxin, chloroquine, doxycycline and amiodarone.
- The concept for loading and maintenance dose is valid also for short $t_{1/2}$ drugs and IV administration in critically ill patients. For example, lidocaine, used for cardiac arrhythmia is given as an IV bolus followed by slow IV infusion or intermittent fractional dosing.

AUTONOMIC NERVOUS SYSTEM

Drug Treatment of Glaucoma

- Glaucoma can be of two types:
  1. Open-angle (wide angle, chronic simple) glaucoma
  2. Angle-closure (narrow angle, acute congestive glaucoma)
- The drug treatment for the above types are as follows:
  - *Open-angle glaucoma*:
    - *Beta adrenergic blockers*: They can be administered topically. They act by reducing aqueous formation, e.g. timolol and betaxolol.
    - *Alpha adrenergic agonists*: They lower intraocular tension by augmenting: uveoscleral outflow or decreasing aqueous production, e.g. dipivefrine and apraclonidine.
    - *Prostaglandin analogs*:They act by increasing permeability of tissues in ciliary muscle or by an action on episcleral vessels, e.g. latanoprost, travoprost and bimatoprost.
    - *Carbonic anhydrase inhibitors*: They limit bicarbonate ion production in ciliary epithelium, e.g. acetazolamide and dorzolamide.
    - *Miotics*: Topical pilocarpine.
  - *Angle-closure glaucoma*:
    - *Hypertonic mannitol*: Infused IV, decongest the eye by osmotic action
    - *Acetazolamide*: 0.5 g IV followed by oral twice daily is started concurrently.
    - *Mitotic*: Once it starts falling, pilocarpine (1–4%) is instilled every 10 minutes initially and then at longer intervals.

  - *Topical beta-blocker*: Timolol 5% is instilled 12 hourly; in addition, apraclonidine (1%) or latanoprost (0.005%) instillation may be added.
- Drugs are given only to terminate the attack.
- Definitive treatment is surgical/laser iridotomy.

Atropine Sulfate: Used in Preanesthetic Medication

- *Justification*
  - To reduce ether induced excessive salivation and tracheal bronchial secretion and thus to reduce the chance of aspiration pneumonia and reflex laryngospasm.
  - To reduce reflex bradycardia during endotracheal intubation and visceral manipulation.
  - To prevent bradycardia and hypotension during repeated injections of succinylcholine.
  - To prevent halothane-induced bradycardia and also halothane-induced cardiac arrhythmias due to sensitization of hearth to epinephrine.

AUTACOIDS

Levocetrizine

- *Identification*:
  - It is 2nd generation antihistaminics.
  - It is active R (-) enantiomer of cetirizine and is effective at half dose.
- *Pharmacological actions*:
  - It has marked affinity for H_1 receptors and penetrates brain poorly → mild sedation, subjective somnolence experienced by many recipients, slightly impairs psychomotor performance.
  - It does not prolong cardiac action potential or produce arrhythmias.
  - It inhibits release of histamines and cytotoxic mediators in the secondary phase of allergic response → thus benefit allergic disorders by other actions as well.
- *Pharamacokinetics*: It attains higher and longer lasting concentrations in the skin → efficacy in urticaria/atopic dermatitis.
- *Indications*: Upper respiratory allergies, pollinosis, urticaria, atopic dermatitis, adjuvant in seasonal asthma produces less sedation.

Aspirin

- *Uses*:
  - As an analgesics
  - As an antipyretics
  - Acute rheumatic fever
  - Rheumatoid arthritis
  - Osteoarthritis
  - Post-AMI
  - Post-stroke
  - *Less common uses are*:
    - Pregnancy-induced hypertension and preeclampsia
    - Patent ductus arteriosus

- Familial colonic polyposis
- Prevention of colon cancer
- Prevent flushing attending nicotinic acid ingestion.

RESPIRATORY SYSTEM

Sodium Cromoglycate

- *Identification*: Mast cell stabilizers and synthetic chromone derivative
- *Mechanism of action*:
  - It blocks calcium influx in mast cells.
  - It inhibits degranulation of mast cells.
  - It restricts release of mediators of asthma like histamine, LTs, PAF, IL, etc.
  - Chemotaxis of inflammatory cells is inhibited.
- *Pharmacokinetics*:
  - Not absorbed orally.
  - Administered as an aerosol through metered dose inhaler
  - Small fraction is absorbed systemically.
  - Rapidly excreted in urine and bile.
- *Uses*:
  - Bronchial asthma—used as a long-term prophylactic in mild-to-moderate asthma.
  - Allergic rhinitis
  - Allergic conjunctivitis.
- *Side effects*: Bronchospasm, throat irritation, cough, etc.

HORMONES

Anabolic Steroids

- *Introduction*: Anabolic steroids promote protein synthesis and increase muscle mass resulting in weight gain.
- Synthetic androgens with greater anabolic activity than androgenic activity.
- *Examples*:
  - *Intramuscular*: Nandrolone and phenylpropionate
  - *Oral*: Oxandrolone, stanozolol and ethylestrenol
  - *Both oral and intramuscular*: Methandienone.
- *Uses*:
  - To improve appetite and feeling of well-being in chronic illness.
  - During recovery from prolonged illness.
  - To counteract catabolic effects of exogenous adrenal cortical hormones.
  - Osteoporosis.
  - To control itching in chronic biliary obstruction.
- *Misuse*: They are often misused by athletes and hence included in "dope test".
- *Side effects*:
  - Virilization in females
  - Edema
  - Growth impairment in children.

Glimepiride

- *Type*: Sulfonylureas group of oral hypoglycemics.
- *Mechanism of action*:
  - *Pancreatic action*:

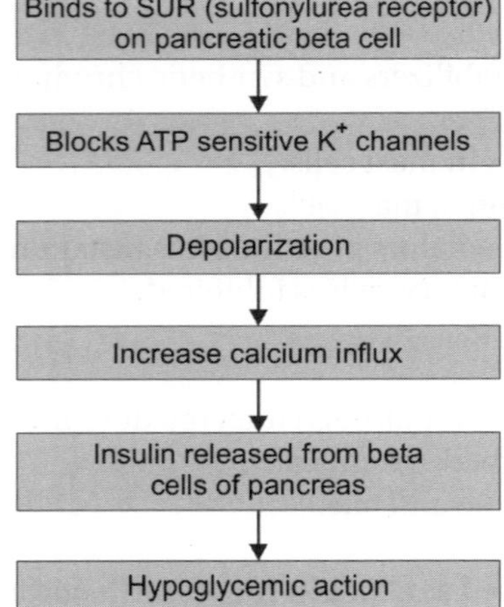

    - Decreased release of glucagon from pancreatic alpha cells to some extent.
  - *Extrapancreatic action*:
    - Decreased hepatic clearance of insulin.
    - Suppression of hepatic gluconeogenesis.
    - Increases number of insulin receptors
    - Increases peripheral tissue sensitivity to insulin.
  - *Pharmacokinetics*:
    - Well absorbed orally
    - 90% more plasma protein bound
    - Low volume of distribution
    - Some are metabolized and produce more active metabolites.
- *Use*: They are used in treatment of NIDDM.
- *Side effects*: Nausea/vomiting, hypoglycemia, paresthesia, weight gain and hypersensitivity.

Emergency Contraceptives

- *Introduction*: These are also called postcoital pill. These are for uses in a woman not taking any contraceptive who had sexual intercourse risking unwanted pregnancy.
- The common standard regimens are:
  - *Levonorgestrel*: 0.75 mg two doses 12 hours apart or 1.5 mg single dose taken as soon as possible but before 72 hours of unprotected intercourse.
  - *Ulipristal*: 30 mg single dose as soon as possible but within 120 hours of intercourse.
  - *Mifepristone*: 600 mg single dose taken within 72 hours of intercourse.
- *Mechanism of action*:
  - Endometrium is either hyperproliferative, hypersecretory or atrophic and in any case "out of phase" with fertilization, i.e. not suitable for nidation.

- Uterine and tubal contractions may be modified to disfavor fertilization.
- It may dislodge a just implanted blastocyst or interfere with fertilization or implantation.

Misoprostol

- *Type*: It is a PGE1 analog. It is a methyl PGE1 ester and a longer-acting synthetic PGE1 derivative.
- *Uses and mechanisms*:
  - *Peptic ulcer*: It inhibits acid output dose dependently. It has a short duration of action (3 hours) and is poorer in relieving ulcer pain.
  - Prevention and treatment of NSAID associated GIT injury and blood loss.
  - *Abortion in early pregnancy*: Used in combination with mifepristone or methotrexate.
  - *Postpartum hemorrhage*: Misoprostol (oral) can be given to control it.
- *Side effects*: Diarrhea, abdominal cramps, uterine bleeding, need for multiple dosing, etc.

PERIPHERAL NERVOUS SYSTEM

Lignocaine

- *Identification*: Immediate potency and duration injectable anesthetic a/k/a lidocaine.
- *Mechanism of action:*
  - Lidocaine traverses the neuronal membrane in its unionized form.
  - It reionizes in the axoplasm.
  - Cationic form of lidocaine binds to the receptor located within the channel in its intracellular half
  - Stabilizes the channel in its inactivated state reduces probability of channel opening.
  - Refer to Figure 26.2; KDT; p. 362.
- *Pharmacological action:*
  - *Nervous system*:
    - *Peripheral nerves*: Order of nerve fibers affected is—autonomic fibers > Pain > Temperature > Touch > Pressure > Motor fibers
  - *Central nervous system (CNS)*:
    - Initially CNS stimulation is followed by CNS depression at higher doses. This causes tremor, excitement, twitching, etc.
    - Large doses can cause respiratory depression, coma and death.
  - *Cardiovascular system (CVS)*:
    - Heart—decreases pacemaker activity, contractility, conductivity, heart rate, cardiac output, etc.

      *Bupivacaine is more cardiotoxic than other lidocaines.
    - Blood vessels—produce hypotension due to vasodilation and myocardial depression.
- *Pharmacokinetics:*
  - High first-pass metabolism and effective orally.
  - Doses must be reduced in liver diseases.
- *Uses:* It is most widely used local anesthetic. It is used for various purposes like:
  - As EMLA (Emetic Mixture of Local Anesthetics- Lignocaine (2.5%) and prilocaine (2.5%)- used for dermal anesthetic during venesection and skin graft.
  - Used in ventricular arrhythmia.

- *Used for*:
  - Surface anesthesia
  - Infiltration anesthesia
  - Nerve block anesthesia
  - Spinal anesthesia
  - Epidural anesthesia
  - Bier's block.
- *Side effects:*
  - *CNS*: Restless, tremors, headache, convulsions, etc.
  - *CVS*: Bradycardia, hypotension, arrhythmias, allergies, etc.
- *Contraindications*:
  - Methemoglobinemia
  - Infants.

CENTRAL NERVOUS SYSTEM

Carbamazepine

- *Introduction*: Carbamazepine is a widely used antiepileptic drug. It is chemically related to imipramine.
- *Uses*:
  - Focal seizures and complex partial seizures (CPS): Most effective drug for CPS.
  - Trigeminal and related neuralgias: In this disease, it is a drug of choice. It benefits by interrupting temporal summation if certain trigger zones in the mouth and face. It is not useful in diabetic, traumatic and other forms of neuropathic pain.
  - Bipolar disorders: Alternative to lithium.
  - Also used in mania.
  - Roland's epilepsy: For this epilepsy, it is a drug of choice.

Propofol

- *Type*: Fast-acting intravenous general anesthetic.
- *Mechanism of action:* Potentiates action of GABA, glycine.
- *Pharmacokinetics*:
  - It is an oily liquid employed as 1% emulsion.
  - Distribution ($t_{1/2}$): 2–4 minutes
  - Elimination ($t_{1/2}$): 100 minutes.
- *Uses*:
  - Used for day care procedures.
  - Used IV for both induction as well as maintenance. Sometimes, it is supplemented by fentanyl and used for total IV anesthesia.
  - It lacks airway irritancy and is preferred in asthmatics.
  - It is suited for outpatient surgery as residual impairment is less marked.
  - It is a drug of choice for sedating intubated patients in intensive care units in subanesthetic doses.
- *Side effects*:
  - It may cause cardiac and respiratory depression.
  - Pain during injection is minimized by combining with lidocaine.

Levodopa

- *Type*: It is an antiparkinsonian drug. It is a precursor of dopamine.
- *Mechanism of action*:

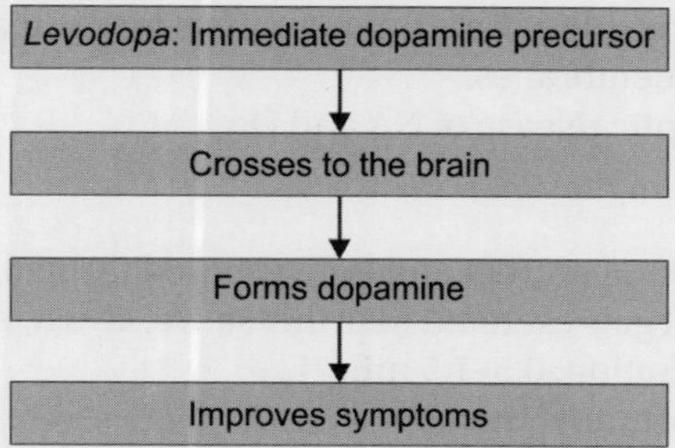

- *Pharmacokinetics*:
  - Rapidly absorbed from small intestine.
  - Bioavailability is affected by–gastric emptying and presence of amino acids in food.
  - High FPM in GI mucosa and liver, only 1% reaches brain.
  - Plasma $t_{1/2}$ is 1–2 hours.
- *Side effects*:
  - At initiation of therapy— nausea and vomiting, postural hypotension, cardiac arrhythmia, exacerbation of angina, alteration in taste sensation.
  - After prolonged therapy—abnormal movement, behavioral effects, fluctuation in motor performance (on-off effect).
- *Cautious use* is needed in elderly, patients with cardiac, hepatic and renal disease, peptic ulcer, glaucoma and gout.
- *Drug interactions*:
  - *Pyridoxine*: It abolishes the therapeutic effect by enhancing its peripheral decarboxylation.
  - *Phenothiazine, butyrophenones, metoclopramide*: They reverse the therapeutic effect of levodopa by blocking DA receptors.
  - *Nonselective MAO inhibitors*: They may cause hypertensive crisis.
  - *Antihypertensive drugs*: Postural hypotension is accentuated.
  - Atropine and some other anticholinergics have additive therapeutic action.

Lithium

- *Identification*: It was the first drug used for treatment of mania. It is a small monovalent cation.
- *Mechanism of action*: In the neuronal membrane—

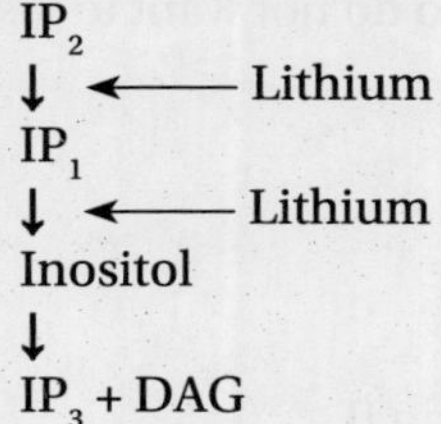

- *Effects*:
  - Lithium inhibits hydrolysis of inositol-1 phosphate by inositol monophosphatase. As a result, release of IP_3 and DAG, which are second messengers for both alpha adrenergic and muscular transmission are reduced.
  - Lithium can mimic the role of Na^+. This may affect ionic fluxes across brain cells or modify property of cellular membranes.
  - It decreases presynaptic release of NA and DA.
- *Pharmacokinetics*:
  - Effective orally
  - Does not bind to plasma protein and is distributed throughout the total body water.
  - Not metabolized and gets excreted in urine, saliva, sweat, etc.
  - Therapeutic concentration: 0.5–1.5 mEq/L.
  - TDM is required for optimal therapy.
- *Uses*:
  - Acute mania
  - Maintenance in bipolar disorder
  - Cluster headache
  - Felty syndrome.
- *Side effects*:
  - Fine tremors
  - *Neurotoxicity*: Coarse tremors
  - Hypothyroidism
  - Polyuria
  - Teratogenic: Ebstein's anomaly in fetus.
- *Contraindication*: Pregnancy.

Dissociative Anesthesia

- *Introduction*: It is characterized by profound analgesia, immobility, amnesia with light sleep.
- *Site of action*: The primary site of action is in the cortex and subcortical areas, not in the reticular activating system, which is the site of action of barbiturates.
- *Effects*:
  - The patient appears to be conscious, i.e. opens his eyes, makes swallowing movements and his muscles are stiff, and he is unable to process sensory stimuli and does not react to them. Thus, the patient appears to be dissociated from his body and surroundings.
  - Respiration is not depressed, bronchodilation, airway reflexes are maintained. Muscle tone is increased. Non-purposive limb movements occur. Heart rate, cardiac output and BP are elevated due to sympathetic stimulation, e.g. ketamine
  - Ketamine has been used for operations on the head and neck in patients who have bleed, in asthmatics (relieves bronchospasm), in those who do not want to lose consciousness and for short operations.

CARDIOVASCULAR SYSTEM

Losartan

- *Type of drug*: It is a competitive antagonist of angiotensin II.

- *Mechanism of action*: It blocks the overt action of all, such as:
  - Vasoconstriction
  - Central and peripheral sympathetic stimulation
  - Release of aldosterone and adrenaline from adrenals
  - Renal action promoting salt and water reabsorption
  - Central action like thirst, vasopressin release and growth promoting action on heart and blood vessels
- No inhibition of angiotensin-converting enzyme (ACE) has been noted.
  - Difference between losartan and other ACE inhibitors:
    - They do not interfere with the degradation of bradykinin and other ACE substrate.
    - They result in more complete inhibition of AT1 receptor activation.
    - They result in indirect AT2 receptor activation.
- *Pharmacokinetics*:
  - Oral absorption is not affected by food.
  - Bioavailability— only 33% due to first-pass metabolism.
  - Metabolized in the liver
  - $t_{1/2}$ is 2 hours.
  - No dose adjustment is required in renal insufficiency. But dose should be reduced in hepatic dysfunction
- *Uses*:
  - One of the first-line antihypertensives
  - Portal hypertension due to cirrhosis
  - Congestive heart failure.
- *Side effects*:
  - Hypotension
  - Hyperkalemia
  - Few reports of cough and angioedema
  - Teratogenic.

Amlodipine

- *Type*: It comes under the dihydropyridines class of calcium channel blockers (CCBs).
- *Mechanism of action*:
  - Amlodipine blocks voltage sensitive L type calcium channels by binding to alpha 1 subunit

    ↓

    Prevents entry of calcium into cell

    ↓

    No excitation–contraction coupling in the heart and vascular smooth muscles as there is delay in recovery of calcium channels
- Amlodipine

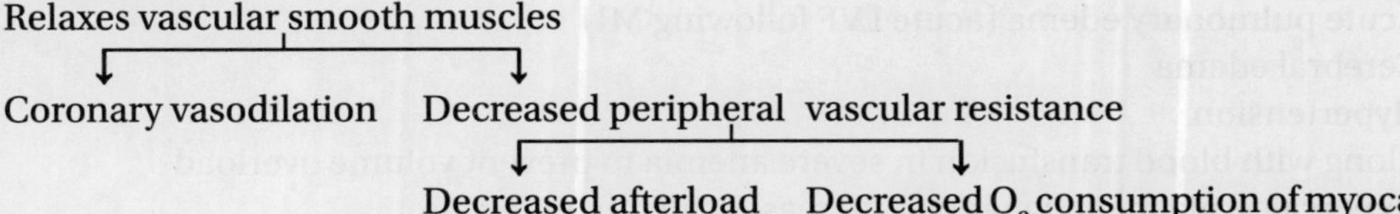

- *Pharmacokinetics*:
  - Absorbed slowly after oral administration
  - High bioavailability
  - Metabolized in liver and excreted in urine.
- *Uses*:
  - Exertional angina
  - Variant angina
  - Unstable angina
  - Hypertension
  - Raynaud's phenomenon.
- *Side effects*:
  - Hypotension
  - Reflex tachycardia
  - Headache and flushing
  - Ankle edema.

RENAL

Furosemide

- *Identification*: High ceiling diuretic
- *Mechanism of action*:
  - *Site of action*: Thick loop of Henle
  - *Mechanism*:
    - Furosemide binds to luminal side of $Na^+K^+2Cl^-$ cotransporter
    - Block $Na^+K^+2Cl^-$ cotransporter
    - Increased excretion of Na^+ and Cl^- in urine
    - Tubular fluid reaching DCT has more Na^+
    - More Na^+K^+ exchange
    - K^+ loss
    - Furosemide has also weak carbonic anhydrase inhibiting activity
    - Increases HCO_3^- and PO_4^{3-} excretion
    - Also increases Ca^{2+} and Mg^{2+} excretion
- *Pharmacokinetics*:
  - Rapidly absorbed from GI
  - Given orally, IV or IM
  - Rapid onset after IV administration
  - Short duration of action (2–4 hours).
- *Uses*:
  - Edema of any etiology—cardiac, hepatic or renal
  - Drug of choice for nephrotic and other forms of resistant edema
  - Acute pulmonary edema (acute LVF following MI)
  - Cerebral edema
  - Hypertension
  - Along with blood transfusion in severe anemia to prevent volume overload
  - Hypercalcemia in malignancy—increases calcium excretion.

- *Side effects:*
  - *Electrolyte problems*:
    - Hypokalemia
    - Hyponatremia
    - Hypokalemic metabolic alkalosis
    - Hypocalcemia and hypomagnesemia
    - Ototoxicity
    - Hypersensitivity.
  - *Metabolic problems*:
    - Hypoglycemia
    - Hyperuricemia
    - Hyperlipidemia
- *Drug interaction*:
  - Furosemide + Digoxin = Causes hypokalemia, may lead to digoxin toxicity
  - Furosemide + Aminoglycoside = Chances of ototoxicity
  - Furosemide + NSAID = NSAID inhibits PG synthesis and blocks PG-mediated hemodynamic changes of loop diuretics.

BLOOD AND BLOOD FORMATION

Low Molecular Weight (LMW) Heparin

- *Introduction*: Heparin has been fractionated into LMW forms (MW = 3000–7000)
- *Mechanism of action*: LMW heparins selectively inhibit factor Xa with little effect on IIa. They act only by inducing conformational change in AT III and not by providing a scaffolding for interaction of AT III with thrombin. So, LMW heparin have smaller effect on aPTT and whole blood clotting time. It has lesser antiplatelet action.Lower incidence of hemorrhagic complications.
- *Pharmacokinetics*: It has many advantages, e.g.
  - Better subcutaneous bioavailability
  - Longer and more consistent $t_{1/2}$
  - Laboratory monitoring not required
  - Lesser risk of osteoporosis.
- *Uses*:
  - Prophylaxis of deep vein thrombosis (DVT) and pulmonary embolism in high-risk patients undergoing surgery, stroke or other immobilized patients.
  - Treatment of DVT
  - Unstable angina and MI
  - Maintains patency of cannula and shunts in dialysis patients.

GASTROINTESTINAL

Ondansetron

- *Type*: It comes under a distinct class of antiemetic drug

- *Mechanism of action*: Ondansetron blocks the depolarizing action of 5HT exerted through $5HT_3$ receptors on vagal afferents in the GIT as well as in NTS and CTZ

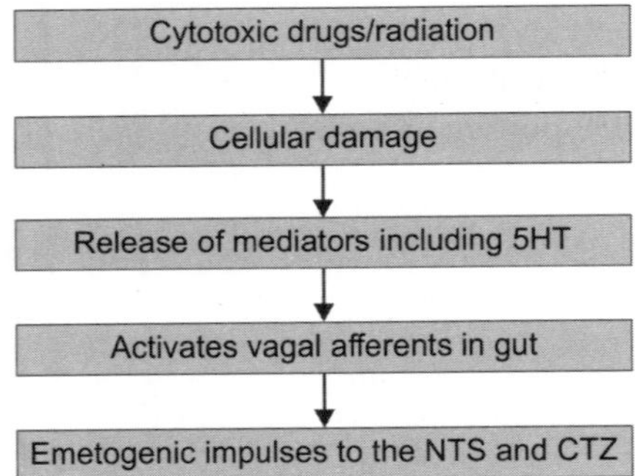

  - Ondansetron blocks emetogenic impulses both at their peripheral origin and their central relay.
  - A weak gastrokinetic action and a minor 5HT4 antagonism has also been shown.
- *Pharmacokinetics*:
  - Oral bioavailability—60–70%
  - Metabolized by hydroxylation, glucuronide and sulfate conjugation.
- *Uses*:
  - Cancer chemotherapy/radiation-induced vomiting
  - Postoperative nausea and vomiting (PONV)
  - Disease/drug-associated vomiting
  - Preanesthetic medication
  - Hyperemesis gravidarum.
- *Drug interactions*: No clinically significant drug interactions are noted.
- *Side effects*:
  - Generally well tolerated
  - Headache and dizziness
  - Mild constipation and abdominal discomfort.

Omeprazole

- *Type*: It is a proton pump inhibitor. It inhibits the final common step in gastric acid secretion
- *Mechanism of action*:

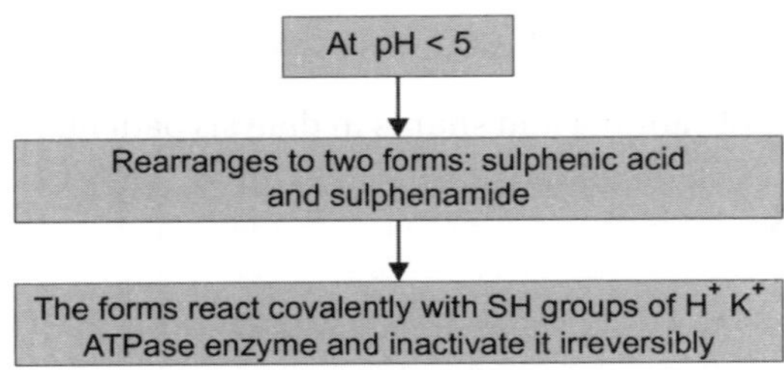

- Omeprazole acts only after absorption into bloodstream and subsequent diffusion into the parietal cell; it gets concentrated in acidic pH of the canaliculi because the charged forms generated there are unable to diffuse back.

- *Pharmacokinetics*:
  - Omeprazole is a HIT and RUN drug: Effect remains long after drug is eliminated from plasma. Action remains for 2–3 days.
  - Bioavailability reduced by food, so it should be taken before meals.
- *Uses*:
  - Peptic ulcer
  - Bleeding peptic ulcer
  - Stress ulcer
  - GERD
  - Zollinger-Ellison syndrome
  - Aspiration pneumonia.
- *Side effects*: Nausea, headache, muscle and joint pains, dizziness complained by 3–5%.
- *Drug interactions*:
  - Omeprazole inhibits oxidation of certain drugs: Diazepam, warfarin, phenytoin levels may increase
  - May interfere with activation of clopidogrel by inhibiting CYP2C19.

ANTIMICROBIALS

Albendazole

- *Identification*: It is an anthelminthic drug.
- *Mechanism of action*: It has a broad-spectrum activity.
  - It binds to beta-tubulin and inhibits microtubule polymerization.
  - It blocks glucose transport into the cell.
  - As a result, intestinal parasites are slowly immobilized and die slowly.
- *Uses*:
  - Highly effective against intestinal nematodes—round worm, hookworm, pin worm, whip worm, thread worm and also mixed worm infestations.
  - Preferred in neurocysticercosis, as it is:
    - Cheaper
    - Shorter duration of treatment
    - Reaches high concentration in the brain and CNS
    - Less toxic and better tolerated.
  - Hydatid disease
  - Filariasis
  - Cutaneous larva migrans
- *Pharmacokinetics*:
  - Given orally
  - Erratic absorption—absorption increased by fatty food
  - Metabolized in liver
  - Active metabolite—albendazole sulfoxide.

- *Side effects*:
  - Rare, well tolerated
  - GI: Nausea, vomiting
  - Few have dizziness.
  - Prolonged use may cause fever, alopecia, jaundice, headache and neutropenia.

Ciprofloxacin

- *Identification*: Most potent first-generation fluoroquinolone active against broad-spectrum bacteria.
- *Mechanism of action*:
  - Ciprofloxacin inhibits
  - DNA Gyrase topoisomerase IV
  - Gram-negative bacteria Gram-positive bacteria
  - Nicking inhibited inhibition of separation of daughter DNA strands
  - Negative supercoils formed
  - Resealing of DNA strands
  - Inhibition of DNA synthesis
  - Bactericidal
- Most susceptible: Aerobic gram-negative bacilli, especially Enterobacteriaceae and *Neisseria*
- Other distinct features:
  - High potency—MBCs close to MICs
  - Long postantibiotic effect on Enterobacteriaceae, *Pseudomonas* and *Staphylococcus*.
  - Low frequency of mutual resistance or plasmid type resistance.
  - Protective microorganisms spared.
  - Less active at acidic pH.
- *Pharmacokinetics*:
  - Rapidly absorbed orally
  - Food delays absorption
  - Good tissue penetrability
  - Excreted primarily in urine
  - Urinary and biliary concentrations are higher than plasma.
- *Side effects*:
  - *GI effects*: Nausea, vomiting, etc.
  - *CNS effects*: Headache, dizziness, etc.
  - Hypersensitivity reactions
  - *Tenosynovitis, tendon rupture*: Athletes are susceptible.
- *Contraindications*:
  - Pregnancy
  - Young children—to present cartilage damage.

Rifampicin

- *Identification*:
  - It is first-line antitubercular drug.
  - It is a derivative of rifamycin.
  - It acts on all types of bacillary subpopulations.

- *Mechanism of action*:
  - Rifampicin binds to beta subunit of DNA dependent RNA polymerase (rPOB gene).
  - It inhibits RNA polymerase.
  - No RNA synthesis.
- *Selective toxicity*: Because mammalian RNA polymerase does not bind rifampicin.
- *Mechanism of resistance*: Mutation in rPOB gene reduces its affinity for the drug.
- *Uses:*
  - Only drug effective against all mycobacteria including *M. leprae* (leprosy)
  - Brucellosis (doxycycline + rifampicin)
  - Legionellosis
  - *Staphylococcus* infections (infective endocarditis, osteomyelitis)
  - Prophylaxis of meningococcal meningitis (*Neisseria meningitidis*) and meningitis caused by *Haemophilus influenzae*.
- *Pharmacokinetics*:
  - Rapidly absorbed from GIT
  - Metabolized in liver
  - Active deacetylated form is excreted in bile and undergoes enterohepatic cycling. Rest excreted in urine.
  - Reduce dose in liver failure patients.
- *Side effects:*
  - Flu syndrome
  - Cutaneous syndrome
  - Abdominal syndrome
  - Acute chest syndrome
  - Hepatotoxic
  - Hemolysis
  - Acute renal failure
  - Acute tubular necrosis
  - Interstitial nephritis
  - Orange discoloration of urine and secretions (harmless).

Azithromycin

- *Identification*: This is a macrolide antibiotic and a semisynthetic congener of erythromycin.
- *Mechanism of action*: Azithromycin binds to bacterial 50S subunit inhibits protein synthesis
- *Spectrum*: Extended spectrum antibacterial, effective against MAC, *Haemophilus influenzae, Salmonella*, Malaria, *Toxoplasma gondii*, etc.
- *Uses:*
  - Drug of choice for—
    - Atypical pneumonia (*M. pneumoniae*)
    - Trachoma (*C. trachomatis*)
    - Chancroid (*H. ducreyi*)
    - Donovanosis (Donovans bacillus granulomatis)
  - *Dosage*: 500 mg OD 1hour before or 2 hours after food for 3–5 days.
- *Pharmacokinetics:*
  - Long acting
  - Good absorption from GI

- Acid stable
- Wide tissue distribution
- Shows concentration-dependent effect (CDE).
- *Drug interactions*: Rare.

Ketoconazole

- *Type*: First orally effective broad spectrum antifungal drug.
- *Mechanism of action*: It impairs ergosterol synthesis by inhibits 14 alpha demethylase enzyme:

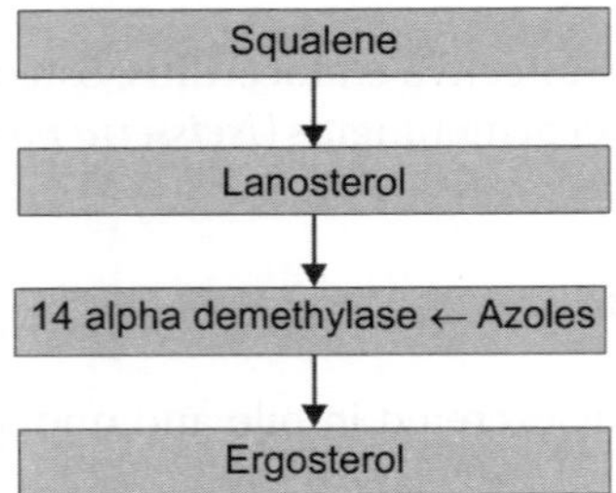

- *Pharmacokinetics*:
  - Orally and topically effective
  - Absorption favored by acidic environment
  - Highly plasma protein bound.
- *Uses*:
  - Dermatophytosis—used topically for *T. pedis, T. cruris, T. corporis* and *T. versicolor*.
  - Candidiasis
  - Kala-azar
  - Dermal leishmaniasis
  - Cushing's syndrome.
- *Side effects*:
  - Most toxic among azoles
  - Anorexia, nausea, vomiting
  - Reduces adrenal cortical steroids synthesis and may cause gynecomastia, loss of libido, impotence in males and menstrual problems in females
  - Hepatotoxicity
  - Hypersensitivity.
- *Drug interactions*: It is an enzyme inhibitor and increases the effect of following drugs by inhibiting their metabolism: sulfonylureas, phenytoin, warfarin, etc.

Meropenem

- *Type*: One of the newer carbapenems
- *Mechanism of* action: It acts by inhibiting bacterial cell wall synthesis and produces bactericidal activity and is active against both gram-positive and gram-negative bacteria, aerobes and anaerobes.
- *Pharmacokinetics*:
  - Injected intravenously
  - Not destroyed by dihydropeptidase and does not require cilastatin

- *Uses*:
  - Reserve drug for treatment of serious nosocomial infections
  - Treatment of infections caused by cephalosporin resistant bacteria
  - Diabetic foot
  - *Pseudomonas* infection- combined with aminoglycosides.
- *Side effects*: Diarrhea, vomiting, skin rashes, hypersensitivity, less likely to cause seizures.

Superinfection

- *Definition*: Appearance of a new infection due to antimicrobial therapy. The causative organism of superinfection should be different from that of the primary disease.
- *Cause*: Mostly due to excessive use of broad spectrum antimicrobials like tetracyclin, chloramphenicol, clindamycin, ampicillin, etc.
- *Mechanism*: The antimicrobials alter the normal bacterial flora as a result of which the host defense mechanism is impaired. Then, pathogens easily invade the host, multiply and produce superinfection.
- *Causative organism*: May be fungi or bacteria
- *Sites involved*: Body cavities having direct communication with exterior, e.g. rectum, oral cavity, vagina, upper respiratory tract, etc.
- *Examples*: Diarrhea (*Candida albicans*) and pseudomembranous colitis (*Clostridium difficile*).
- *Predisposing factors*:
  - Immunocompromised
  - Diabetes
  - Malignancy.
- *Precautions*:
  - Use of specific antimicrobials
  - Use of probiotics
  - Avoiding unnecessary use of antimicrobials.

Chloroquine

- *Type*: It is a rapidly acting erythrocyte schizonticide against all species of *Plasmodium*.
- *Mechanism of action*:

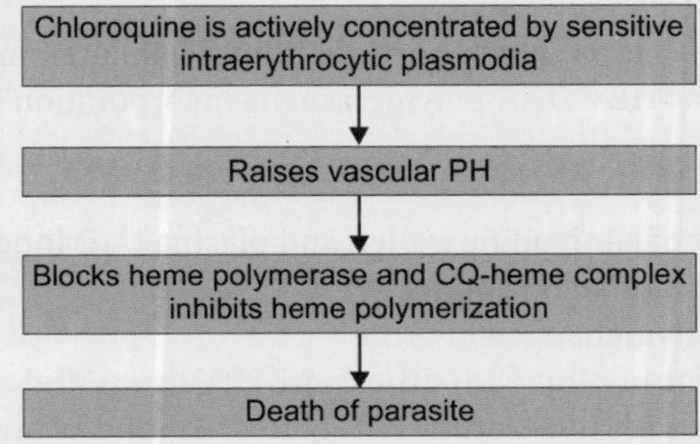

- It has anti-inflammatory, local irritant, local anesthetic, weak muscle relaxant, antihistaminic and antiarrhythmic properties too.
- *Mechanism of resistance*: Efflux of chloroquine with help of the *P. falciparum* chloroquine resistance transporter (PfCRT) and the *P. falciparum* multidrug resistance (PfMDR) is also implicated.
- *Pharmacokinetics*:
  - Oral absorption is good.
  - About 90% plasma protein bound
  - It has high affinity for nuclear chromatin.
  - Its selective accumulation in retina is responsible for ocular toxicity.
  - Partly metabolized in liver
  - Slowly excreted in urine
  - $t_{1/2}$ is 3–10 days or more.
- *Use*:
  - Chloroquine is the drug of choice for clinical cure and suppressive prophylaxis of all types of malaria except that caused by resistant *Plasmodium*.
  - Rheumatoid arthritis
  - Extraintestinal amebiasis
  - Discoid lupus erythematosus (DLE)
  - Lepra reaction and photogenic reactions
  - Infectious mononucleosis
  - Photogenic reactions
  - Systemic lupus erythematosus (SLE).
- *Other actions*: It is active against *E. histolytica* and *Giardia lamblia* too.
- *Mnemonics*: RED LIPS
- *Side effects*:
  - Nausea, vomiting, anorexia, itching, headache, etc.
  - Parenteral administration causes hypotension, cardiac depression, arrhythmia and CNS toxicity.
  - Prolonged use of high dose causes loss of vision due to retinal damage.
  - Loss of hearing, photo allergy, mental disturbances, myopathy and graying of hair
  - No abortifacient or teratogenicity reported.

Lamivudine

- *Identification*: It is a doxycycline analog.
- *Mechanism of action*: It is phosphorylated intracellularly and inhibits HIV release transcriptase as well as HBV DNA polymerase. Its incorporation into DNA results in chain termination.
- *Pharmacokinetics*:
  - Oral bioavailability of lamivudine is high and plasma $t_{1/2}$ is longer (6–8 hours).
  - Intracellular $t_{1/2}$ is more than12 hours.
  - It is mainly excreted unchanged in urine
- *Uses*: It is used in combination with other anti-HIV drugs and appears to be as effective as AZT. It synergizes with most other NRTIs for HIV and is an essential component of

all first- line triple drug NACO regimens for AIDS. It is also a first-line drug for chronic hepatitis.

- *Side effects*:
  - Generally, well tolerated and has low toxicity.
  - Headache, fatigue, rashes, nausea, anorexia, abdominal pain, pancreatitis and neuropathy (rare).

Amikacin

- *Identification*: It is an aminoglycoside antibiotic used to treat different types of bactericidal infections. It is a semisynthetic derivative of kanamycin. It is on the WHO list of "Essential drugs".
- *Mechanism of action*: It can be described in two main stages—
  - Transport of the aminoglycoside through the bacterial cell wall and cytoplasmic membrane: Diffuse across the outer coat of gram-negative bacteria through porin channels. Entry from the periplasmic space across the cytoplasmic membrane is carrier mediated which is linked to the ETC. The penetration is dependent on maintenance of a polarized membrane and is an oxygen dependent active process.
  - After entry, binding to the ribosomes resulting in inhibition of protein synthesis as shown below:

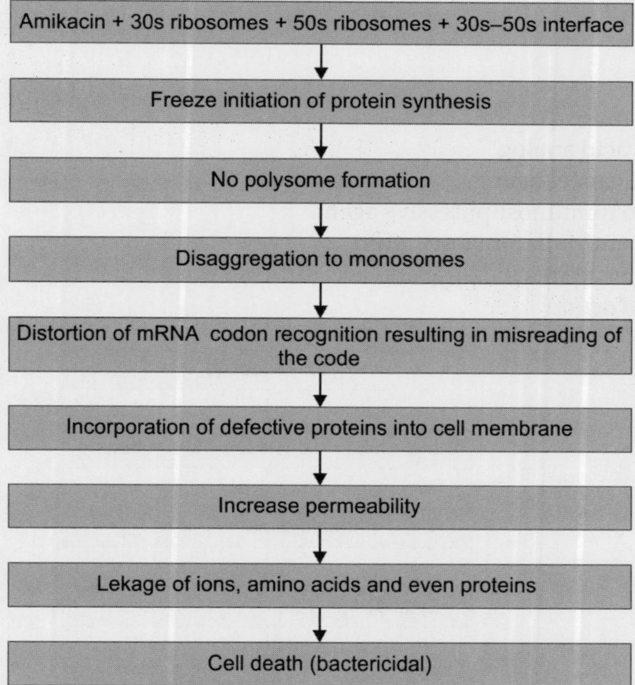

- *Mechanism of resistance*: It has a wide spectrum of activity since it is resistance due to:
  - Mutation decreasing the affinity of ribosomal proteins that normally bind the aminoglycoside.
  - Decreases efficiency of the aminoglycoside transporting mechanism.

- *Side effects*:
  - Ototoxicity—cochlear damage and vestibular damage
  - Nephrotoxicity.
- *Pharmacokinetics*:
  - Highly ionized and neither absorbed nor destroyed in the gut.
  - Absorption from injection site in muscles is rapid.
  - Distributed only extracellularly, so Vd is nearly equal to ECF volume.
  - Cross placenta and can be found in fetal blood and amniotic fluid.
  - Not metabolized in body and excreted unchanged in urine.
  - Plasma $t_{1/2}$ is 2–4 hours.
- *Uses*:
  - Hospital acquired gram-negative bacillary infection where gentamicin/tobramycin resistance is high
  - Used for multidrug resistant-tuberculosis (MDR-TB)
  - Respiratory tract infection in critically ill patients
  - *Pseudomonas, Proteus* or *Klebsiella* infections
  - Meningitis caused by gram-negative bacilli
  - Subacute bacterial endocarditis (SABE).

CHEMOTHERAPY

Methotrexate

- *Type and features*:
  - It is a folic acid analog.
  - It is an anticancer agent.
  - It is also an immunosuppressive agent.
  - It has also anti-inflammatory effects.
  - It is a cell-cycle specific drug and acts during S phase.
- *Mechanism of action*:

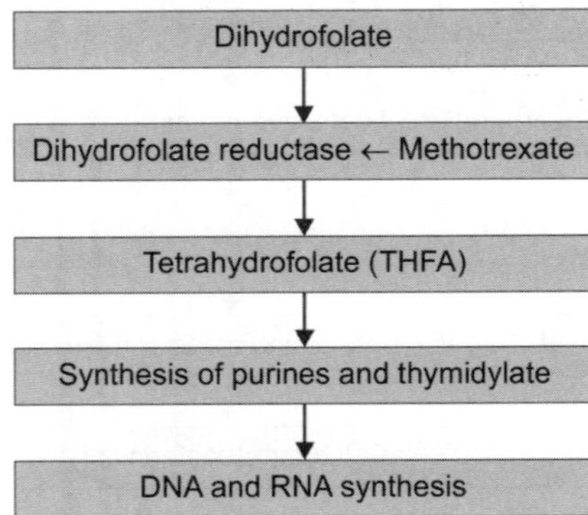

  - Methotrexate is a competitive inhibitor of dihydrofolate reductase.
  - It depletes intracellular THFA which is required for synthesis of purines and thymidylate, which in turn, are required for DNA and RNA synthesis.

- *Pharmacokinectics*:
  - Well absorbed orally
  - Can be given IM, IV or intrathecally.
- *Uses*:
  - Drug of combination for choriocarcinoma
  - Used in acute leukemia, Burkitt's lymphoma and breast cancer
  - Rheumatoid arthritis
  - Inflammatory bowel disease
  - Organ transplantations
  - Psoriasis.
- *Side effects*:
  - *General toxicity*: Bone marrow suppression, alopecia and GI problems.
  - *Other effects*: Megaloblastic anemia, pancytopenia and hepatic fibrosis
- *Drug interactions*:
  - Salicylates, tertracyclines displace methotrexate bound to plasma proteins and increase its free form in plasma leading to toxicity.
  - NSAIDs and sulfonamides— potentiates methotrexate toxicity by interfering with its excretion.

MISCELLANEOUS MEDICATIONS

Interferon Alpha

- *Introduction*: Interferons (IFNs) are species specific but disease non-specific low molecular weight cytokines secreted from cells infected with a virus or intracellular parasite.
- *Sources*: Pooled leukocytes (alpha IFN), fibroblasts (beta IFN) or activated T cells (gamma IFN).
- *Mechanism of action*: Interferons bind to specific cell surface receptors and affect viral replication at multiple steps, viz.
  - Viral penetration
  - Synthesis of viral mRNA
  - Assembly of viral particles and their release
  - Direct or indirect suppression of viral protein synthesis, i.e inhibition of translation:

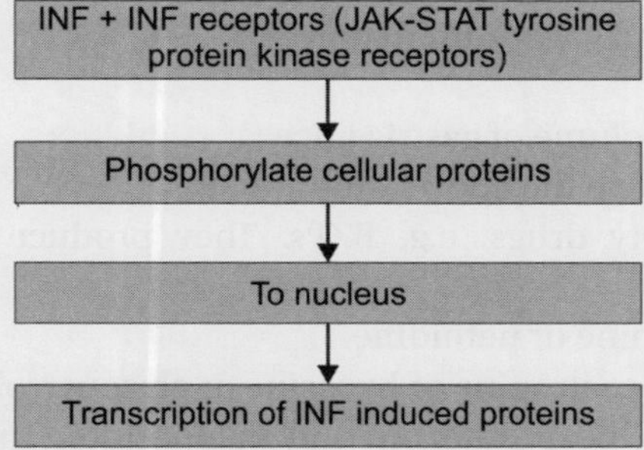

- *Types*: IFN alpha, beta and gamma.

  - Only IFN alpha 2A and 2B produced by recombinant technology are available and are clinically used.
  - Their PEGylated forms are mostly used. Plasma levels of peg IFN alpha 2A are sustained twice longer than those of peg IFN alpha 2B.
- *Pharmacokinetics*:
  - IM/SC injection
  - Degrades mainly in liver and kidney.
  - Remains detectable in plasma for 24 hours.
  - INF is generally administered thrice weekly as cellular effects are longer lasting because INF-induced proteins persist.
  - Complexed with polyethylene glycol (PEG IFN).
  - Orally not effective.
- *Uses*:
  - Chronic hepatitis
  - AIDS-related Kaposi's sarcoma
  - Condyloma acuminata
  - Chronic myeloid leukemia
  - Follicular lymphoma
  - Cutaneous T-cell lymphoma
  - Multiple myeloma.
- *Side effects*:
  - Flu like symptoms—fatigue, aches, malaise, fever, anorexia, etc.
  - Neurotoxicity—numbness, neuropathy, tremor, altered behavior, etc.
  - Myelosuppression—dose-dependent neutropenia and thrombocytopenia
  - Thyroid dysfunction
  - Hypotension, transient arrhythmia, alopecia and liver dysfunction.

Preanesthetic Medication

- *Definition*: Preanesthetic medication refers to the use of drugs before anesthesia to make it more pleasant and safe.
- *Aims*:
  - Relief of anxiety and apprehension
  - Amnesia
  - Supplement analgesic action
  - Decrease secretions and vagal stimulation
  - Antiemetic
  - Decrease acidity and volume of gastric juice
  - The drugs used to achieve the above are—
    - Sedative antianxiety drugs, e.g. BZPs. They produce tranquility and smoothen induction.
    - Opioids, e.g. morphine or pethidine
    - Anticholinergics, e.g. atropine or hyoscine or glycopyrrolate
    - Neuroleptics, e.g. chlorpromazine and haloperidol. They allay anxiety, smoothen induction and have antiemetic action.

- H_2 blocker/PPIs, e.g. ranitidine and pantoprazole
- Antiemetics, e.g. metoclopramide, domperidone and ondansetron.

Antisnake Venom

- *Introduction*: Antisnake venom (ASV) may be monovalent for a specific type of snake or polyvalent for four common poisonous snakes like Indian spectacle cobra, common krait, Russel's viper and saw-scaled viper. In India, the monovalent type is not available.
- *Preparation*:
  - It is prepared by hyperimmunization of horse against a particular venom or common four venoms.
  - It is produced in both liquid and lyophilized form.
- *Storage*:
  - Lyophilized and powdered ASV requires to be kept cool (>25°C) and last for 5 years.
  - 1 vial of 10 mL ASV is meant for neutralizing 6 mg of Russell's viper venom, cobra venom and 4.5 mg of common krait and saw-scaled viper venom.
- *Indications*: Signs of local envenomation like swelling, blister, necrosis, systemic bleeding, prolonged clotting time, etc.
- *Dose*: Following initial dose is recommended—10 vials at time for both neurotoxic and hemotoxic envenomation.
- *Other important features are*:
  - No prior skin test for anaphylaxis required.
  - ASV can neutralize the circulating toxin, not the toxin already fixed in tissue.
  - Helpful within 4 hours of bite, action is doubtful beyond 24 hours.

CHAPTER

6

Explain Why and Mechanism of Action

Avishek Layek, Dyuti Deepta Rano, Tathagata Bhattacharya

GENERAL PHARMACOLOGY

1. In clinical practice, why is efficacy of a drug more important than its potency? Explain.

- Drug potency refers to the amount of drug needed to produce a certain response.
- Drug efficacy refers to the maximum response that can be elicited by a drug.
  In clinical practice, efficacy becomes more decisive factor in choosing a drug because:
  - Higher potency does not confer superiority unless the potency of the therapeutic effect is selectively increases over potency of adverse reactions.
  - A higher efficacious drug produces a level of pharmaceutical effect not attainable by any amount of a low efficacy drug (e.g. morphine can produce a level of analgesia which cannot be attained by any dose of paracetamol).
  - Depending on the type of drug, both higher efficacy (as in case of furosemide conferring utility for mobilizing edema fluid in renal failure) or lower efficacy (in case of diazepam conferring safety in overdose) could be clinically advantageous.

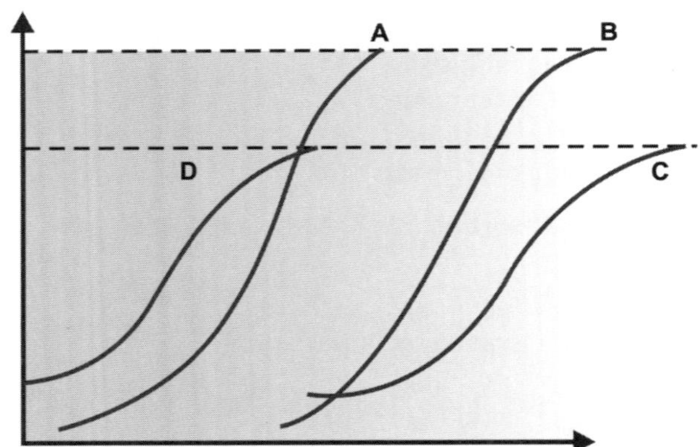

Fig. 6.1: Interpretation of Log dose response curve as shown
(i) B is less potent but equally efficacious as A; (ii) C is less potent and less efficacious than A;
(iii) D is most potent; but less efficacious then A and B and equally efficacious as C

2. Why is therapeutic drug monitoring (TDM) essential for certain drugs? Explain.

- *Principle of TDM*: C_{PSS} of a drug depends on F,V, CL
  [C_{PSS}, steady-state plasma concentration; F, fraction reaching systemic circulation; V, volume of distribution; CL, clearance]

- Due to individual variations in these 3 parameters, the actual plasma concentration in a patient may be 3 to 1/3rd times of average population data
- Hence, following TDM; revised dose rate

$$= \frac{\text{Previous dose rate} \times \text{Target } C_{PSS}}{\text{Measured } C_{PSS}}$$

- Measured C_{PSS} is calculated following drug administration.

- TDM is particularly useful in following cases:
  - Drugs with low safety margin—increase in C_{PSS} might be dangerous like digoxin or lithium.
  - If individual variation is large for a specific drug like antidepressants.
  - If there is failure of therapy without apparent reason, as in in antimicrobials
- TDM is never used for drugs whose response can be clinically assessed like any drug which is used for slowing the heart rate can be assessed by pulse rate measurement.

3. Why is inhalational route preferred over systemic route for drug delivery for bronchial asthma? Explain.

- Four classes of antiasthmatic drugs are available for inhalational use:
  1. β_2-agonist
  2. Anticholinergics
  3. Chromoglycate
  4. Glucocorticoid.
- These antiasthmatic drugs are preferred for inhalational route over systemic route because:
  - Lower dose is needed as inhalational route directly delivers drug to the site of action.
  - Systemic side effects are lowered.
  - Faster onset of action is achieved over oral administration.
  - Metered dose inhalers help in dose actuation.
  - May be self-administered with practice.
  - More than one drug may be nebulized together in emergencies.
  - Less chance of suppression of HPA axis.

4. Why are basic drugs better absorbed in alkaline media and acidic drugs in acidic media? Explain.

- Most drugs are weak electrolytes, i.e. their ionization is pH dependent.
- The ionization of weak acid A is given by the equation:

$$pH = pKa + \log [A^-]/[HA] \text{ (Henderson–Hasselbalch equation)}$$

- So, weakly acidic drugs, e.g. sodium phenobarbitone, sodium sulfadiazine, etc. ionize more at alkaline pH and weakly basic drugs like atropine sulfate, chloroquine phosphate, etc. ionize more at acidic pH and 1 scale change in pH causes 10-fold change in ionization.
- Ions, being lipid-insoluble, do not diffuse across cell membrane. So, acidic drugs in acidic pH and basic drugs in basic pH mostly remain unionized.

5. Why is oral route mostly preferred for drug administration? Explain.

- Oral route is most common and easily available route for drug administration.
- Dosage forms are tablet, capsule, syrup, mixture, spansule, etc.

- The advantages are:
  - It is safer
  - Convenient for repeated and prolonged use
  - Can be self administered
  - Noninvasive
  - Painless
  - Medication need not to be sterile
  - Cheaper
  - Patient compliance is better.

6. Why does ephedrine cause tachyphylaxis? Explain.

- Tachyphylaxis refers to rapid development of tolerance, where doses of a drug repeated in quick succession results in marked reduction in response.
- Tachyphylaxis is usually seen with drugs acting indirectly like ephedrine.
- This drug act by releasing catecholamines in the body, synthesis of which is unable to cope up with the rate of release; resulting in stores being depleted.
- Other mechanisms include:
  - Slow dissociation of the drug from the receptor
  - Desensitization/internalization of the receptor
  - Compensatory hemostatic adaptation.

DRUGS ACTING ON AUTONOMIC NERVOUS SYSTEM

7. Explain mechanism of action of latanoprost in glaucoma.

- *Pathophysiology:*

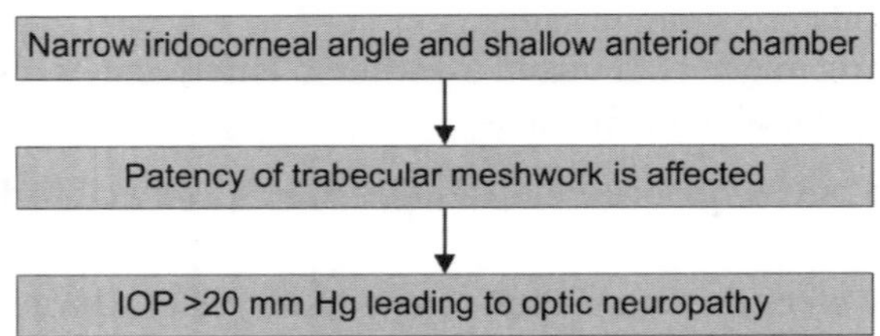

- Latanoprost (PGF_2-alpha analog) increases uveoscleral outflow, which is otherwise a very minor contributor to aqueous drainage by the following mechanisms:
  - Increased permeability of ciliary muscle tissue
  - Action on episcleral vessels
- Also, there is some increase in trabecular outflow.
- Thus, the aqueous drainage is facilitated by mainly by uveo-scleral outflow increase and to little extent also by increase of trabecular outflow.
- Ciliary body COX-2 enzyme has been found to be downregulated in open-angle glaucoma. Hence, low concentration of PGF-2α analog is found to be helpful without inducing inflammation; since COX produced PG analogs.

8. Explain mechanism of action of tamsulosin in benign hypertrophy of prostate (BHP).

In BHP, there is resistance to flow of urine due to increased resistance of large prostate.

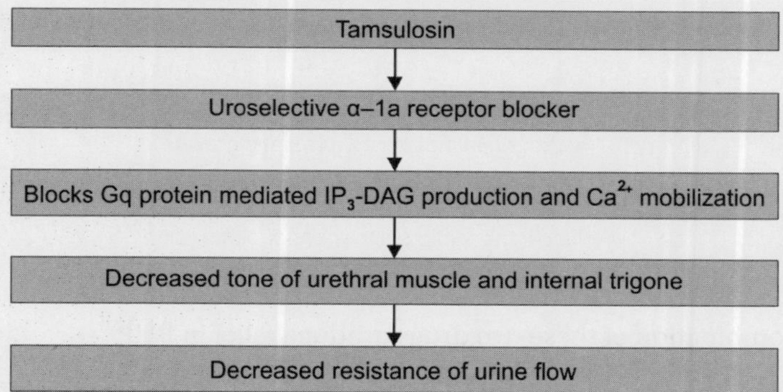

9. Why should beta-blockers not be withdrawn abruptly? Explain.

- Withdrawal of beta-blockers after chronic use should always be gradual otherwise it may lead to the following:
  - Rebound hypertension
  - Worsening of angina
  - Sudden cardiac death.
- This is due to supersensitivity and up-regulation of beta receptors occurring as a result of long-term reduction in agonist stimulation.

10. Why are tamsulosin and finasteride used together in BHP? Explain.

- Benign hypertrophy of prostate leads to increased frequency of micturition and inability to void the bladder completely due to:
  - Enlarged prostate producing outflow obstruction due to fibromusculoglandular proliferation and ball valve action—static component of obstruction.
  - Smooth muscle contraction around the urethra producing obstruction—dynamic component of obstruction.
- Tamsulosin being an alpha1A blocker (uroselective, since alpha1A subtype predominates in bladder base and prostate

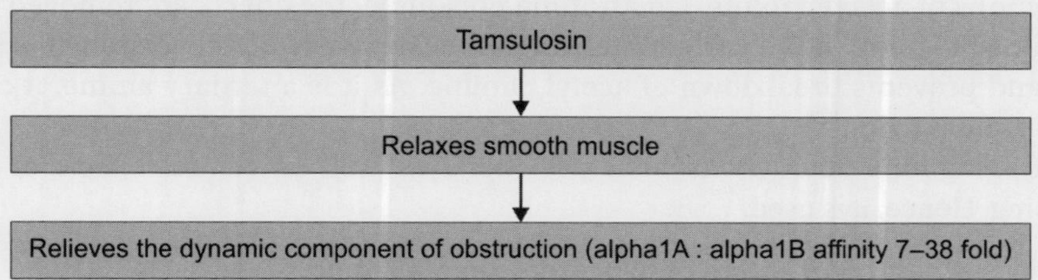

- Finasteride is a competitive inhibitor of enzyme 5-alpha-reductase which converts testosterone to active DHT (dihydrotestosterone) (selective for type 2 isoenzyme, predominant in male urogenital tract).

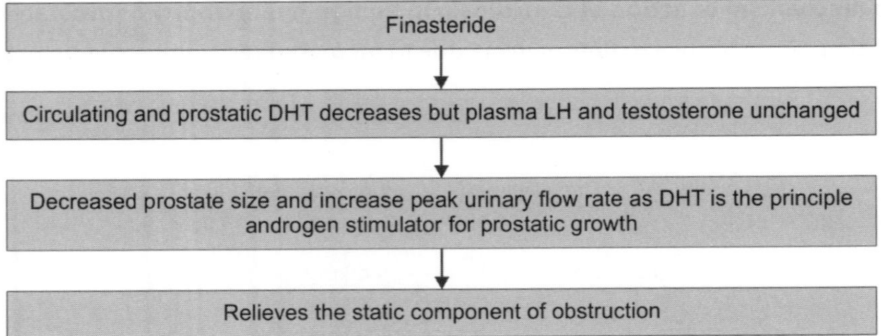

- Therefore, combination of these two drugs produce relief in BHP.

11. Why should oximes be administered within 24 hours of OP poisoning? Explain.

- Oximes are used to restore neuromuscular transmission in case of organophosphate poisoning.
- Oximes has a positively charged quaternary nitrogen which attaches to the anionic site, and oxime end reacts with phosphorus atom attached to the esteratic site. The oxime phosphate so formed diffuses away leaving the reactivated cholinesterase. But oximes should be administered within 24 hours of OP poisoning as the phosphorylated enzyme may undergo an aging by loss of one of the alkyl group and becomes totally resistant to hydrolysis. To prevent this, oxime should be administered as early as possible.

12. Why is neostigmine but not physostigmine used in myasthenia gravis? Explain.

- Neostigmine and physostigmine both are anticholinesterases. By inhibiting cholinesterase, both increase acetyl choline concentration in NMJ. Physostigmine is a tertiary amine and neostigmine is a quaternary ammonium compound. Because of structural similarity with ACh, neostigmine also directly stimulate N_M receptors at NMJ.
- Thus, it improves muscle power in patients with myasthenia gravis. So, neostigmine is preferred.

13. Explain mechanism of action of physostigmine in datura poisoning.

- Atropine is the prototype antimuscarinic drug which blocks muscarinic receptor mediated actions of acetyl choline. On atropine poisoning, the effects are removed by physostigmine (1–4 mg). It is a carbamate anticholinesterase which reversibly block the enzyme and prevents breakdown of acetyl choline. As it is a tertiary amine, it can cross blood-brain barrier.
- So, physostigmine counteracts both peripheral as well as central effects of atropine poisoning. Hence, it is used.

14. Explain mechanism of action of pilocarpine in glaucoma.

Pilocarpine being a cholinomimetic alkaloid directly acts on M3 receptors of sphincter pupillae and ciliary muscle.

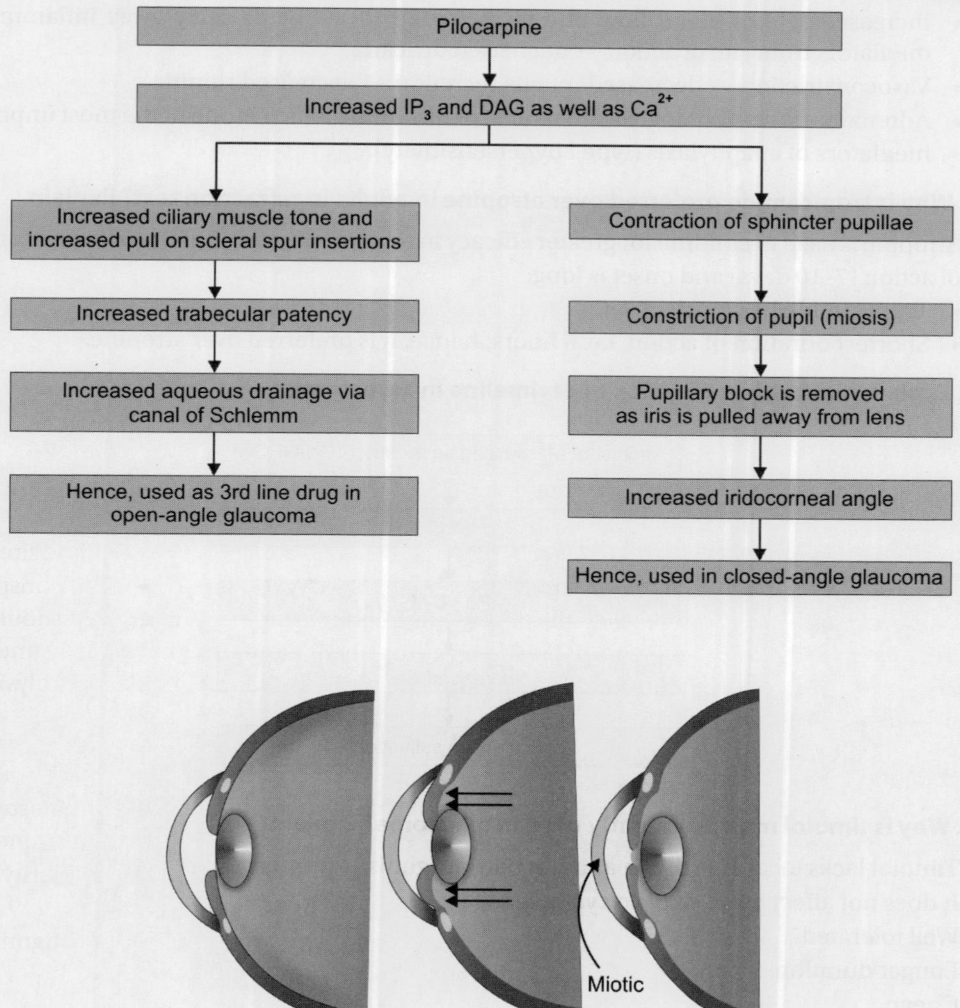

Fig. 6.2: Angle closure glaucoma and its reversal by miotics

15. Explain mechanism of action of adrenaline in acute anaphylactic reaction.

- Anaphylactic reaction is characterized by (i) hypotension, (ii) bronchospasm, (iii) angioedema, (iv) rhinitis, (v) urticaria, etc.
- In such case adrenaline acts as a lifesaving drug (0.3–0.5 mL in 1:1000 dilution (IM) and helps reverse the manifestation by:
  - α_1, β_1-mediated rise of blood pressure
  - β_2-mediated bronchodilation
  - α_1-mediated vasoconstriction → decreased blood flow → decrease edema

- Increased rate of blood flow due to increased BP → helps carry away inflammatory mediators from site of action → decreased urticaria
- Vasoconstriction → decreased mucus secretion → decreased rhinitis
- Adrenaline is a physiological antagonist of histamine which is one of the most important mediators of anaphylaxis (type I hypersensitivity).

16. Why is tropicamide preferred over atropine in adults in refraction test? Explain.

- Atropine is used in children for greater efficacy in refraction testing but it has longer duration of action (7–10 days) and onset is long.
  - Tropicamide has quick onset
  - Shortest duration of action, i.e. 6 hours; hence, it is preferred over atropine.

17. Explain mechanism of action of cevimeline in xerostomia.

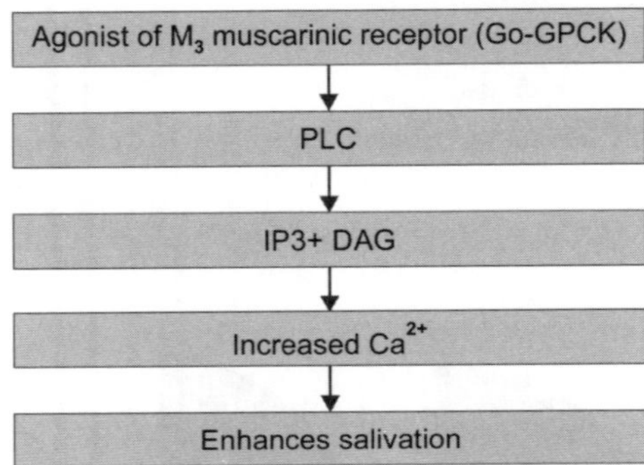

18. Why is timolol most frequently used in glaucoma? Explain.

- Timolol lacks local anesthesia and has partial agonistic property.
- It does not affect pupil size/no cycloplegia.
- Well tolerated
- Longer duration of action
- Cheap
- β_1-selective, no central side effects.

19. Why is propranolol used in thyrotoxicosis? Explain.

- Thyrotoxicosis is an emergency due to decompensated hyperthyroidism.
- Propranolol being a non-selective β blocker is used as:
  - Helps counteract the effects due to sympathetic overactivity and provides immediate symptomatic relief-palpitation, nervousness, tremor, severe myopathy, sweating
  - Decreased peripheral conversion of T_4 to T_3
  - *Dose*: 1–2 mg slow IV followed by 40–80 mg oral QID.

20. Why are β-blockers contraindicated in peripheral vascular disease? Explain.

Non-selective β-blocker → block β_2 vasodilatory receptor → unopposed α_1-mediated vasospasm α worsening of prognosis.

AUTACOIDS AND RELATED DRUGS

21. Explain mechanism of action of sumatriptan in migraine.

- Pathogenesis of migraine is as follows:
  - *Vascular theory*: Initial vasoconstriction and shunting produce cerebral ischemia, and attack is induced. Followed by dilation of vessels and pulsatile contraction leading to pulsatile headache.
  - *Neurogenic theory*:
    - Spreading depression and cortical electrical activity followed by vascular phenomenon.
    - Neurogenic inflammation of blood vessel wall is amplified by release of mediators like 5-HT, neurokinin, substance P, etc.
- Sumatriptan, being a 5-$HT_{1b/1d}$ receptor agonist which is a presynaptic autoreceptor, decreases 5-HT release causing following actions:
  - Constricts dilated cranial blood vessels
  - Constricts dilated arteriovenous shunt in carotid artery
  - Inhibits release of inflammatory neuropeptide
  - Decreased extravasation of plasma proteins across the vessels.

22. Explain mechanism of action of misoprostol.

- Inhibit acid secretion
- Increased HCO_3 secretion
- Increased mucus secretion
- Decreased gastrin secretion
- Increased mucosal blood flow
- Ill-defined cytoprotective role.

23. Explain mechanism of action of aspirin as an antipyretic.

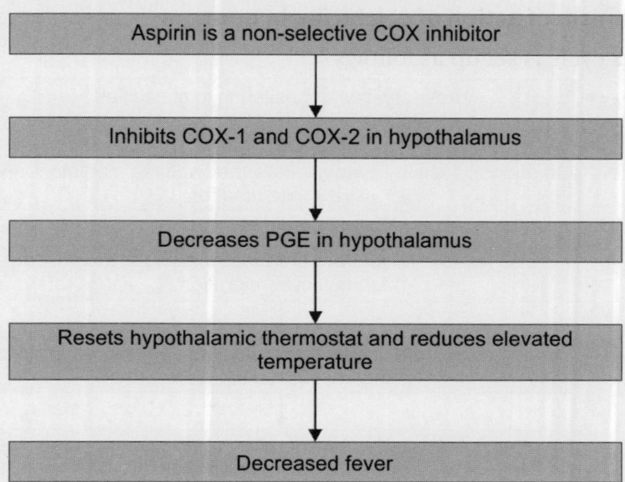

24. Explain mechanism of action of indomethacin in treatment of patent ductus arteriosus.

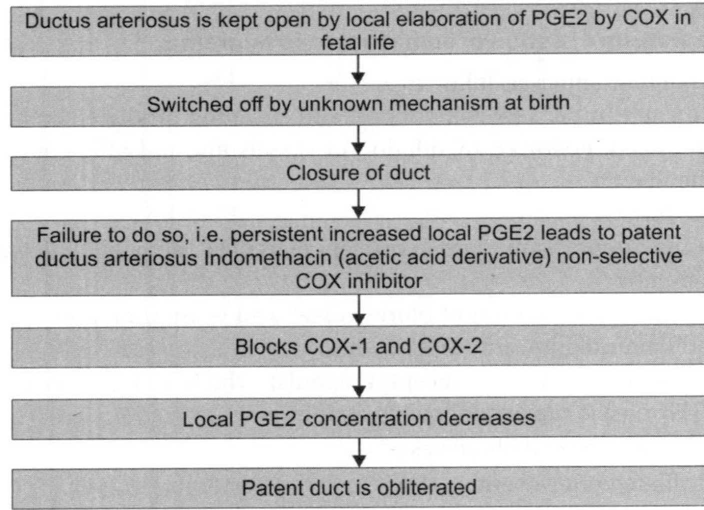

25. Explain mechanism of action of indomethacin in gout.

- It is useful for prophylaxis and treatment of acute and chronic gout.
- It decreases inflammation of joints by:
  - Inhibition of PG synthesis by COX-1 and COX-2 synthesis
  - Also decreases other mediators like bradykinin, histamine, serotonin and inhibits granulocyte adherence
  - Stabilizes lysosomal membrane
  - Inhibition of chemotaxis
  - T-cell function modification
  - Analgesic effect by peripheral COX inhibition, hence useful in acute attack of relieving pain.

26. Explain mechanism of action of colchicine in gout.

- In gout a vicious cycle is set up as follows:

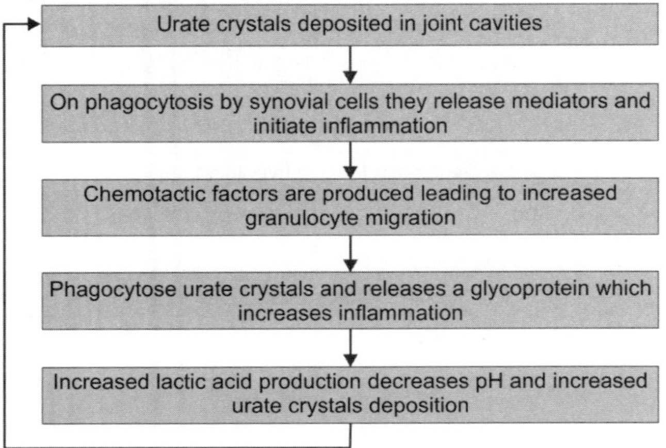

- Colchicine binds to fibrillar protein tubulin and inhibits granulocyte migration, thereby disrupting the vicious cycle by metaphase arrest.

27. Explain mechanism of action of N-acetyl cysteine in paracetamol poisoning.

- Paracetamol poisoning occurs especially in premature children who have low hepatic glucuronide conjugating ability and in alcoholics.
- Mechanism of toxicity is as follows:

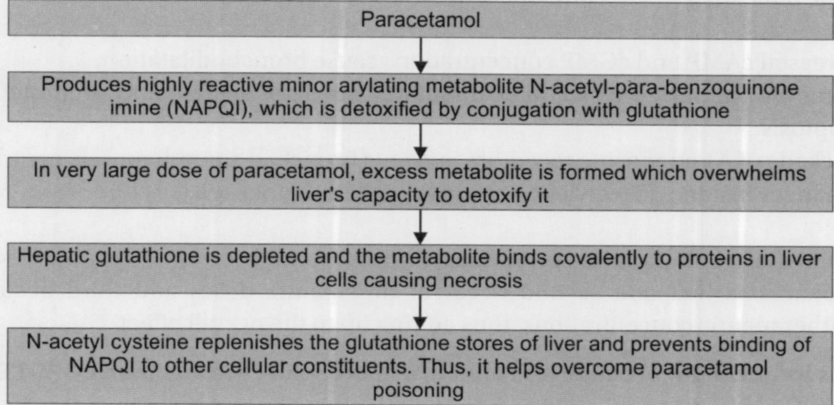

RESPIRATORY SYSTEM DRUGS

28. Explain mechanism of action of corticosteroids in bronchial asthma.

- Bronchial asthma is a disease of the respiratory system with different etiologies but with two constant components:
  - Inflammation and hypersensitivity of the airways
  - Reversible airway obstruction.
- Benefits of using corticosteroids in bronchial asthma are both in treatment of exacerbations and prophylaxis, and they are as follows:
  - Reduce bronchial hypersensitivity
  - Reduce the frequency and severity of exacerbations of bronchial asthma
  - Suppress the response to Ag:Ab reaction and to other stimuli
  - Improve air flow and influence airway remodeling, thus retarding disease progression
  - Increase responsiveness and reverse refractoriness to beta-2 agonists
- Mechanisms of action which produce the above effects are:

Anti-inflammatory actions	*Immunosuppressant actions*
• Induction of annexins in macrophages, endothelium and fibroblast • Negative regulation of COX-2 • Negative regulation of genes for cytokines in macrophages, endothelial cells and lymphocytes • ↓ production of acute phase reactants from macrophages and endothelial cells • ↓ production of ELAM-1 and ICAM-1 in endothelial cells • ↓ expression of transcription factors AP-1, NF-kB • ↓ production of collagenase and stromelysin	• Annexins inhibit phospholipase A_2 → decreased production of PGs, LTs and PAF • ↓ inducible PG production • ↓ production of IL-1, IL-2, IL-3, IL-6, TNFα, GM-CSF, γ interferon fibroblast proliferation and t-lymphocyte function are suppressed, chemotaxis interfered. • Complement function is interfered • Adhesion and localization of leukocytes is interfered. • ↓ histone acetylation • ↓ MAP kinase • Prevention of tissue destruction

29. Explain mechanism of action of theophylline in bronchial asthma.

- Theophylline is a naturally occurring methyl xanthene alkaloid which is useful mainly in acute exacerbations of bronchial asthma.
- There are three different mechanisms of theophylline which are exerted at different concentrations:
  - Mainly selective phosphodiesterase inhibition-4 (PDE-4) which degrades intracellular cyclic nucleotides like cAMP or cGMP

    ↓

    Increased cAMP and cGMP concentrations cause bronchodilatation.

    Moreover, the raised cAMP also attenuates mediator release and promote eosinophil apoptosis.
  - Blockade of A1 adenosine receptors prevents bronchial smooth muscle contraction.
  - Enhances histone deacetylation in airway inflammatory cells

    ↓

    Suppress proinflammatory gene transcription.

    Mechanisms first and second occur at therapeutic doses and third occurs even at subtherapeutic concentrations, thus adding up to the overall effect.

30. Why is ipratropium bromide less effective in bronchial asthma than COPD? Explain.

- Ipratropium bromide is a competitive inhibitor of M_3 muscarnic receptor which is present on bronchial smooth muscle and thus following two effects are obvious:
  1. Decreased or prevention of bronchoconstriction
  2. Decreased tracheal-bronchial secretion

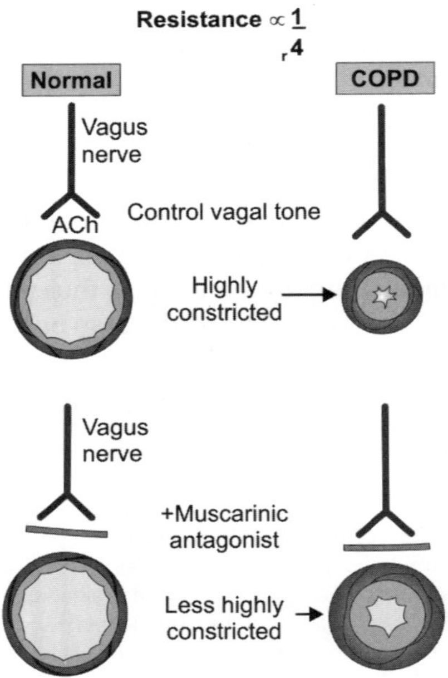

Fig. 6.3: MOA of Ipratropium bromide in COPD

- It is more effective in COPD:
  - In COPD patients, the relief of bronchoconstriction is more pronounced because airways are structurally narrowed and have higher resistant to airflow.
  - Non-neuronal ACh acting on muscarinic (M_3) receptors not innervated by cholinergic nerves may be the cause of structural narrowing. Ipratropium bromide can prevent it too.
  - Vagal tone although not necessarily increased in all cases of COPD, may be the only reversible element of airway obstruction and one that is exaggerated by geometric factors in the narrow airways of COPD. Anticholinergics have an inhibitory effect on vagal tone.
  - Anticholinergics decrease air trapping and improved exercise tolerance in COPD patients.
- It is less effective in bronchial asthma because:
  - Anticholinergics will only inhibit reflex ACh-mediated bronchoconstriction and have no blocking effect on the direct effects of inflammatory mediators, i.e. histamine, leukotriene on bronchial smooth muscles. The latter is the main pathology of bronchoconstriction of bronchial asthma.
  - Anticholinergics have little or no effect on mast cells, microvascular leak or chronic inflammatory response and thus have no effect on inflammatory pathology of bronchial asthma.
  - Inhaled anticholinergics have slower onset of action and so are never used alone in acute exacerbation of bronchial asthma.

31. Explain mechanism of action of salbutamol in bronchial asthma.

- Chain of action is:

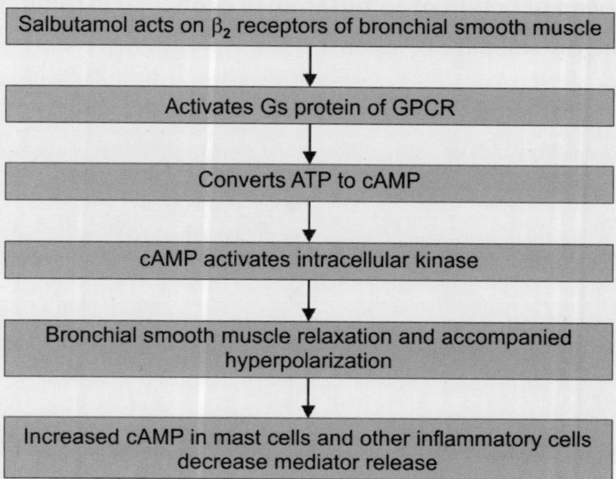

- Mainly relaxes bronchiolar smooth muscle but not large airways.

32. Explain mechanism of action of theophylline in bronchial asthma.

- Theophylline acts by:
  - Inhibition of phosphodiesterase → increased cGMP and cAMP → bronchodilation, vasodilation, cardiac stimulation
  - Blockade of adenosine receptor → reverse of bronchial smooth muscle contraction produced by adenosine (low dose)

- Increased cAMP in inflammatory cells → decreased mediator release and eosinophil apoptosis (first and third in high dose)
- Theophylline (subtherapeutic dose) enhance histone deacetylation in airway inflammatory cells → suppress proinflammatory gene transcription
- Raised of Ca^{2+} from sarcoplasmic reticulum (supratherapeutic).

33. Why is sodium chromoglycate not used in bronchial asthma? Explain.

- It decreases release of asthma mediators like histamine, leukotrienes, PAF, interleukins, etc. and hence used in chronic asthma or prophylaxis.
- It is not used in acute attack because:
  - It is not a bronchodilator.
  - It does not antagonize constrictor action of histamine, acetyl choline and leukotrienes which are already released.

34. Why are inhaled corticosteroids used in asthma but not during acute attack? Explain.

- Peak effects of corticosteroids are seen after 4–7 days of initiating therapy. Hence, they have no role in acute attack.
- They are used in chronic therapy because they:
  - Suppress bronchial inflammation
  - Increase peak expiratory flow rate
  - Prevent episode of acute asthma
  - Reduce need for rescue β_2 agonist inhalation.

35. Explain mechanism of action of salbutamol in bronchial asthma.

- Salbutamol is a highly selective β_2 agonist.
- Its chain of action is:

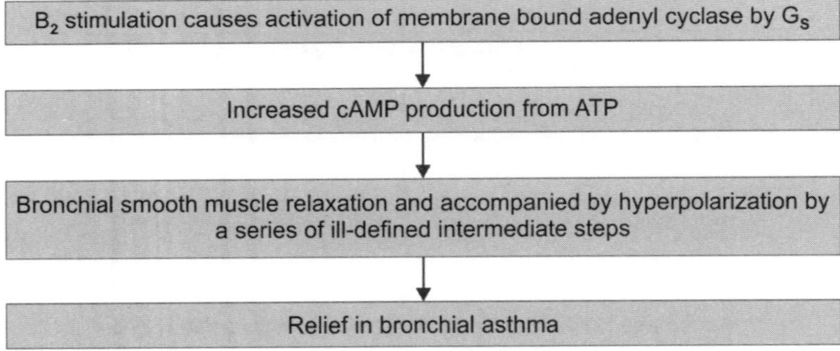

36. May D-tubocurarine produce bronchial asthma? Explain.

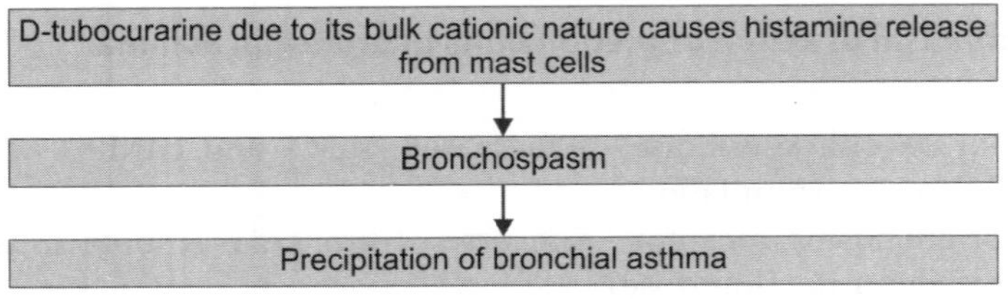

37. Why is montelukast used in prophylaxis of asthma and not in acute attacks? Explain.

- LT C4–D4 are important immunological inflammatory modulators of bronchial asthma.
- Montelukast being competitive antagonist at cysteine-LT-1 receptor brings about the following changes:
  - Decreases cysteine-LT-1 receptor mediated bronchoconstriction
  - Decreases mucous secretion
  - Decreases vascular permeability
  - Decreases eosinophil recruitment
  - Decreases bronchial inflammation and hyperactivity
  - Has additive effect with inhaled steroids, hence permit reduction in steroid dose
  - Even higher additive effect with long acting beta-2 agonist.
- Other advantages are:
  - Very safe adverse effect profile
  - Allowed for use in children <6 years
  - Very few instances of headache and rashes
  - Oral formulation available, hence easier to self administer than as inhalers and cheaper.
- Reason for not using in acute asthma:
  - Low efficacy as no effect in already released inflammatory mediators, hence ineffective in acute exacerbation.
  - Orally administered, no IV or inhaled preparation, hence:
    - Onset of action is slower.
    - Local concentration in respiratory tract is inadequate and erratic.

HORMONES AND RELATED DRUGS

38. Explain mechanism of action of metformin in type 2 diabetes mellitus (T2DM).

- Metformin or biguanides does not cause insulin release but presence of insulin is essential for its action.
- Metformin is not effective in pancreatomized animals and T1DM.
- It activates AMP-dependent protein kinase (AMPK) to play a crucial role in mediating the actions of metformin. The key features of which are:
  - Suppress hepatic gluconeogenesis and glucose output from the liver. This is the main action for lowering blood glucose in diabetics.
  - Enhances insulin-mediated glucose uptake and disposal in skeletal muscle and fat. Insulin resistance in T2DM is thus overcome. This is caused by:
    - Glycogen storage in skeletal muscle
    - Reduced lipogenesis and enhanced fatty acid oxidation in adipose tissue.
  - Interferences with mitochondrial respiratory chain and promotes peripheral glucose utilization through anaerobic glycolysis.
- Metformin also interferes with intestinal absorption of glucose, other hexoses, amino acids and vitamin B_{12}.

39. Explain mechanism of action of teriparatide in osteoporosis.

- Teriparatide is the recombinant preparation of 1–34 residues of amino terminal of human PTH has been recently introduced for the treatment of severe osteoporosis.
- Teriparatide is the only agent that stimulates bone formation.

- It duplicates all actions of PTH, so there is:
  - Increased bone formation
  - Increased calcium resorption in the distal tubule and provides time to time regulation of calcium excretion. It also tends to supplement the hypercalcemic effect by prompting phosphate excretion.
  - Increased calcium absorption from intestine indirectly enhancing formation of calcitriol in the kidney by activating 1-alpha-hydroxylase. Thus, it reduces vertebral as well as nonvertebral features in osteoporotic women as well as men.

40. Explain mechanism of action of pioglitazone (thiazolidinedione).

- Pioglitazone/rosiglitazone is a selective agonist of PPAR-γ (peroxisome proliferator-activated receptor-γ).
- Binds to nuclear PPAR-γ (mainly in fat cell, adipose tissue and other cells).
- Enhances transcription of several insulin responsive genes that regulate carbohydrate and lipid metabolism.
- Sensitizes peripheral tissues to insulin.
- Decrease blood glucose by:
  - Reversing insulin resistance by enhancing GLUT-4 expression and transformation, so entry of glucose in muscle and adipose tissue is improved.
  - Hepatic gluconeogenesis is suppressed.
  - Activation of genes which regulates fatty acid metabolism, thus increases lipogenesis in adipose tissue.
  - Decreased lipolysis and plasma fatty acid level.
  - Also decrease serum TG level and raises HDL level without much change in LDL level by acting on PPAR-α inducing reverse cholesterol transporter and apoproteins.
    [DPP-4 expressed on luminal capillary endothelial cells of gut mucosa, kidney, liver and immune cells.]

41. Explain mechanism of action of DPP-4 inhibitors in T2DM.

- Dipeptidyl peptidase-4 inhibitors
- Competitively and selectively inhibit DPP-4
- Potentiates and increases plasma level of glucagon-like peptide-1(GLP-1) [from L-cells in distal ileum and colon] and glucose-dependent insulinotropic polypeptide (GIP) [enteroendocrine K cells of small bowel].
- Boosts postprandial insulin release, decrease insulin secretion and decrease mealtime as well as fasting blood glucose in T2DM.

42. Explain mechanism of action of acarbose.

- Acarbose is a complex oligopolysaccharide.
- Reversibly inhibits α-glucosidase, the final enzyme for digestion of carbohydrate in brush border in small intestine mucosa.
- Slows down and decreases digestion and absorption of polysaccharide and sucrose
- Postprandial glycemia is reduced without significance increase in insulin level.
- It also promotes GLP-1 release which boosts insulin release → decrease glucagon secretion and mealtime as well as fasting blood glucose in T2DM.

43. Explain mechanism of action of chlorpropamide.

- Chlorpropamide act as:

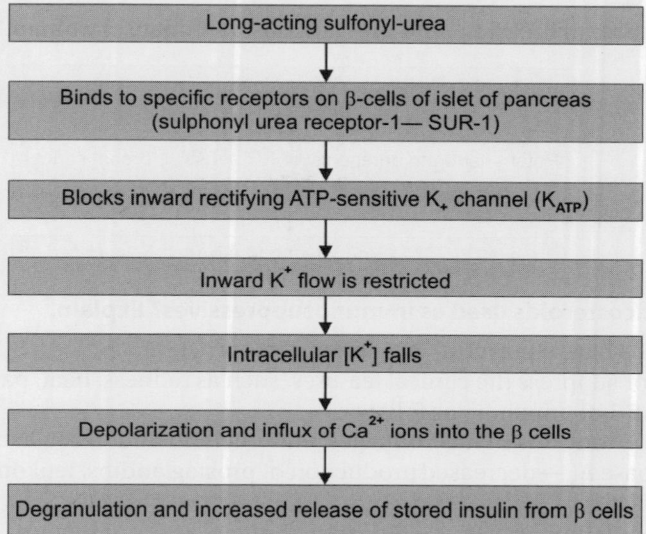

- After few months of administration, the insulinemic action of sulfonylurea are reduced probably due to down regulation of SUR-1 receptor on β-cell but improvement of glucose is maintained by:
  - Increased sensitivity of peripheral tissues (specially liver) to insulin by increasing insulin receptors
  - Release of glucagon.

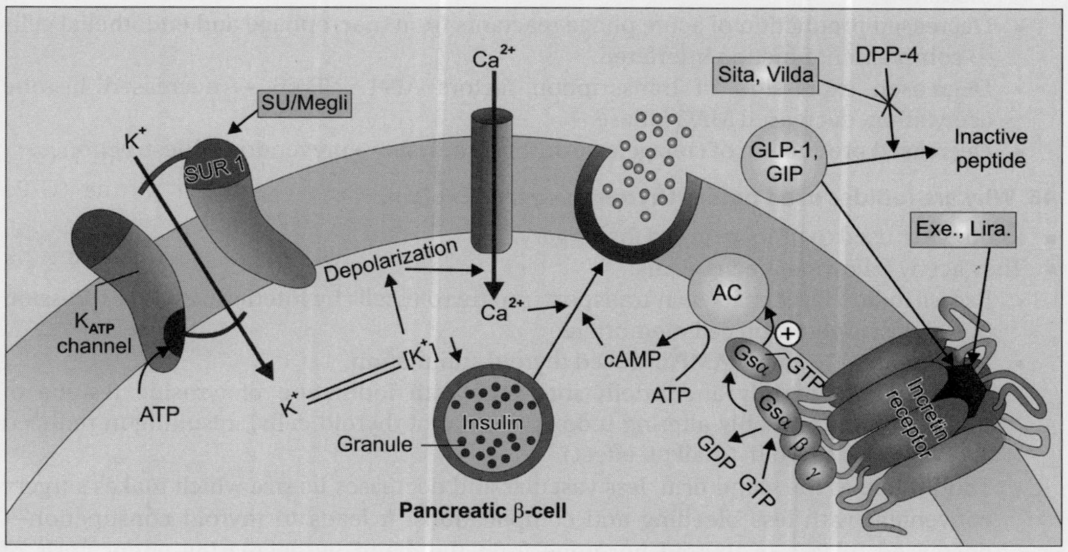

Fig. 6.4: MOA of insulin secretagogues at pancreatic beta-cell level

44. Explain mechanism of action of tamoxifen in breast cancer.

- Tamoxifen is a non-steroidal compound with a selective Estrogen Receptor modulating effect.
- It is used in cancer of breast in both pre- and postmenopausal women.

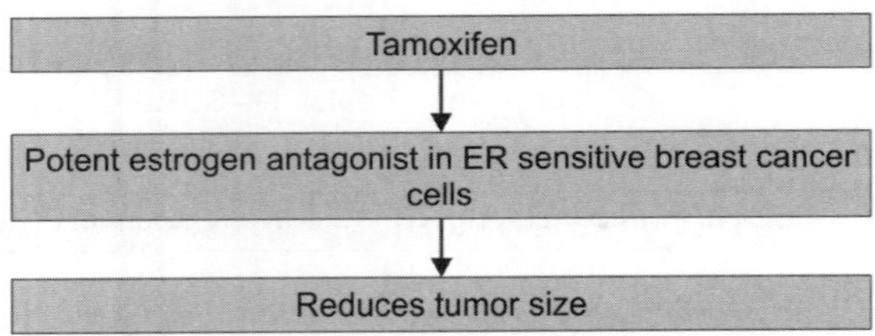

45. Why are corticosteroids used as immunosuppressives? Explain.

- Glucocorticoids have a powerful anti-inflammatory action.
- They prevent or suppress the clinical features, such as redness, heat, pain and swelling.
- They act as anti-inflammatory as follows:
  - Induction of annexins in macrophages, endothelium and fibroblasts. Annexins inhibits phospholipase A_2 → decreased production of prostaglandins, leukotrienes, and platelet-activating factor.
  - Negative regulation of COX-2 → decrease inducible PG production
  - Negative regulation of genes for cytokines in macrophages, endothelial cells and lymphocytes → decrease production of IL-1, IL-2, IL-3, IL-6, TNF-α, GM-CSF → chemotaxis interfered.
  - Decreased production of ELAM-1, ICAM-1 in endothelial cells → adhesion and localization of leukocytes is hampered.
  - Glucocorticoids stabilize the lysosomal membrane and prevent release of inflammatory mediators.
  - Decreased production of acute phage reactants from macrophage and endothelial cells → complement function interfered.
  - Decreased expression of transcription factors AP-1, NF-κβ → decreased histone acetylation, decreased MAO kinase.
  - Decreased production of collagenase and stromolysin → prevention of destruction.

46. Why are iodides used before thyroid surgery? Explain.

- Iodides are used to prepare gland for surgery.
- They act by following mechanisms:
  - Excess iodide inhibits its own transport into thyroid cells by interfering with expression of Na^+–I^+ symporter on cell membrane.
  - It attenuates TSH and cAMP induced thyroid stimulation.
  - Excess iodide rapidly and briefly interferes with iodination of tyrosine residue of thyroglobulin (probably altering redox potential of thyroid cells), resulting in reduced T_3/T_4 synthesis (Wolff–Chaikoff effect).
  - Thus, it makes the gland firm, less vascular and decreases its size which makes surgery convenient with less bleeding and complications. It leads to thyroid constipation→ decreased release of thyroid hormone from the gland by decreasing endocytosis of colloid/proteolysis.

47. Explain mechanism of action of carbimazole in hyperthyroidism.

- Carbimazole is a antithyroid drug.
- It binds to thyroid peroxidase and prevents oxidation of iodide. Thus, the following events occur:
  - It inhibits iodination of tyrosine residue of thyroglobulin.
  - It inhibits coupling of MIT and DIT to form T_3 or T_4.
  - It inhibits oxidation of iodide to iodine.
- Thus, thyroid colloid is depleted over time and blood levels of T_3/T_4 are progressively lowered.

48. Explain mechanism of action of propylthiouracil in hyperthyroidism.

- Propylthiouracil is an antithyroid drug.
- It binds to thyroid peroxidase and prevents oxidation of iodide. Thus, the following events occur:
  - It inhibits iodination of tyrosine residue of thyroglobulin.
  - It inhibits coupling of MIT and DIT to form T_3 or T_4.
  - It inhibits oxidation of iodide to iodine.
  - Inhibits peripheral conversion of T_4 to T_3 by D_1 type 5'-deiodinase but not by D_2 type.
- Thus, thyroid colloid is depleted over time and blood levels of T_3/T_4 are progressively lowered.

49. Explain mechanism of action of clomiphene citrate in inducing ovulation.

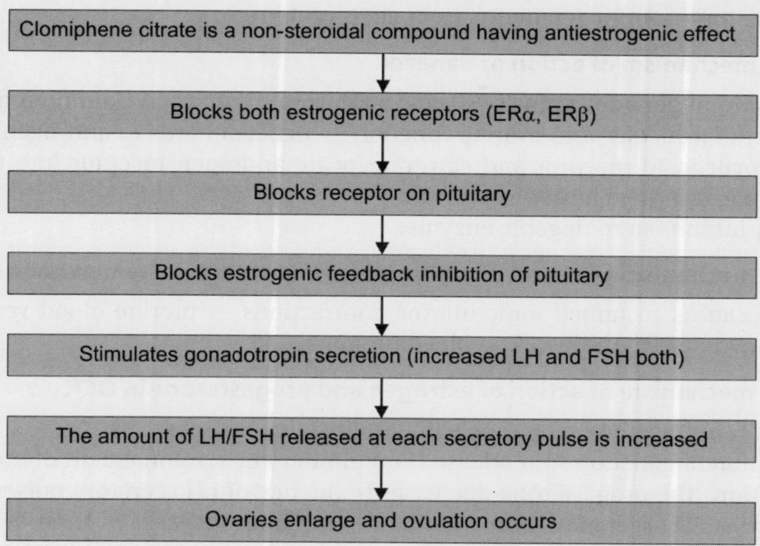

50. Why is oxytocin used in induction of labor and preferred over ergotamine? Explain.

- Synthetic oxytocin (syntocin) is the drug of choice for induction of labor.
- Action of oxytocin on myometrium is independent of innervation.
- Oxytocin binds to special G protein coupled receptor on myometrium. This leads to:
  - Depolarization of muscle fibers and influx of Ca^{2+} ions.

- Generation of IP3 from PIP2 and IP3 mediated intracellular release of Ca^{2+} ions.
- Increased production of PGs by endometrium

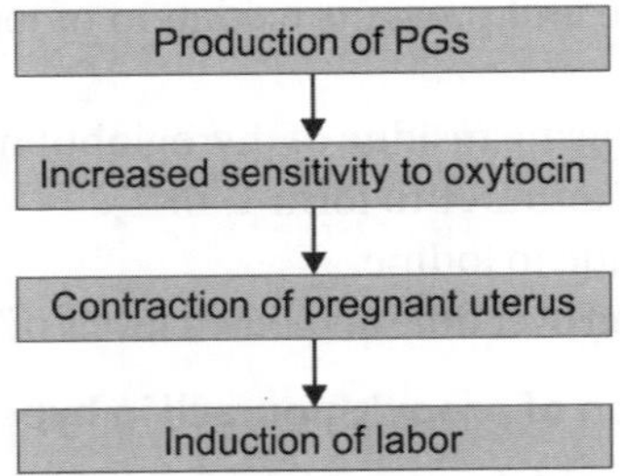

- It is preferred over ergometrine, because:
  - It has short plasma half-life. The intensity of action can be controlled by slow IV infusion and action can be terminated quickly by stopping the drip.
  - At low concentration, there is period of complete relaxation between successive uterine contractions that allow refilling of placental blood vessels by maternal arterial blood and prevent fetal asphyxia.
  - Lower uterine segment is not contracted, so the fetal descent is not compromised.
  - Ergotamine stimulates both uterine segments to contract. At low doses, contractions are rhythmic with a period of relaxation in-between, but at higher doses, the contractions are more powerful and raising the resting tone and the uterus passes into a state of sustained contraction—uterine tetany. So, oxytocin is preferred.

51. Explain mechanism of action of danazol.

- Suppression of gonadotropins (FSH and LH) from pituitary in both men and women → inhibition of testicular and ovarian function → danazol binds to androgen, progesterone and glucocorticoid receptor and can translocate androgen receptor into the nucleus to initiate androgen specific RNA synthesis.
- It directly inhibits steroidogenic enzymes.

52. Explain mechanism of action of ergotamine in postpartum hemorrhage (PPH).

Ergotamine causes sustained tonic uterine contractions → uterine blood vessels are compressed by myometrial meshwork → bleeding stops.

53. Explain mechanism of action of estrogen and progesterone in OCP.

- Hormonal contraceptives interfere with fertility in many ways:
  - Inhibition of gonadotropin release from pituitary by reinforcement of normal feedback inhibition. The progesterone decreases frequency of LH secretory pulses and estrogen decreases FSH secretion, both synergies to inhibit midcycle LH surge. When combined pill is taken both FSH and LH are reduced and midcycle surge is abolished → anovulatory cycle.
  - Thick cervical mucus secretion hostile to sperm penetration is evoked by progestin secretion.
  - Even if ovulation and fertilization occur, the blastocyst may fail to implant, because endometrium is either hypoproliferative or hypersecretory or atrophic → out of phase fertilization.

- Uterine and tubal contractions may be modified to disfavor fertilization.
- The postcoital pill may dislodge just implanted blastocyst.

54. Why is propylthiouracil preferred over carbimazole in pregnancy? Explain.

- In case of pregnancy, the use of antithyroid drugs carries potential risk of fetal hypothyroidism and goiter.
- Propylthiouracil has greater plasma protein binding action than carbimazole which causes less transfer to fetus.
- Thus, propylthiouracil is preferred over carbimazole.

55. Why are progestins added to estrogens in hormone replacement therapy (HRT)? Explain.

- Due to cessation of ovarian function at menopause, women suffer from a number of physical, psychological and emotional consequences for which a combination HRT (estrogen and progestin) is indicated.
- In postmenopausal women, continuous estrogenic stimulation increases the risk of dysfunctional uterine bleeding.
- Progestin is added to counteract the risk of endometrial cancer.

56. Why is hydrochlorothiazide used with triamterene in treatment of chronic hypertension? Explain.

- Hydrochlorothiazide is a thiazide diuretic used in the treatment of uncomplicated hypertension.
- Triamterene is a non-steroidal inhibitor of renal epithelial sodium channel which is a potassium-sparing diuretic.
  - Chronic use of hydrochlorothiazide causes hypokalemia which is manifested as weakness, fatigue, muscle cramps, cardiac arrhythmias, etc. To overcome this, triamterene is coadministered.
  - In addition to this, triamterene also augments the natriuretic response of thiazides.
  - Antihypertensive action of hydrochlorothiazide is also supplemented.

57. Explain mechanism of action of GLP-1 analog.

- GLP-1 analog induces insulin release from pancreatic β-cells.
- It slows gastric emptying.
- It inhibits glucagon release from α-cells.
- It suppresses appetite by activating specific GLP-1 receptor, which is cell surface receptor on β and α-cells, central and peripheral nerves, and gastrointestinal mucosa.

58. Why are prostaglandin (PG) analogs used in 2nd trimester of medical termination of pregnancy (MTP)? Explain.

- Various PG analogs are used in 2nd trimester of MTP, because:
  - PGE_2 and $PGF_{2\alpha}$ uniformly contract human uterus in vivo in pregnant state.
  - Sensitivity to PG is higher in pregnancy for uterus whereas uterus is nor sensitive to oxytocin in early stages of pregnancy.
  - Administration of PG analogs convert oxytocin resistant midterm uterus to oxytocin responsive.

DRUGS ACTING ON PERIPHERAL NERVOUS SYSTEM

59. Explain mechanism of action of succinylcholine used as a muscle relaxant.

Succinylcholine is a depolarizing neuromuscular blocker. It actions are as follows:

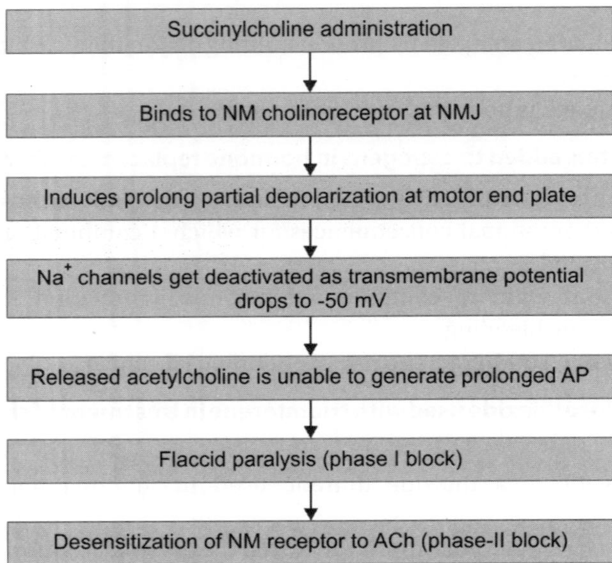

DRUGS ACTING ON CENTRAL NERVOUS SYSTEM

60. Why is methadone used in morphine withdrawal? Explain.

- Methadone is a synthetic opioid, chemically dissimilar but pharmacologically very similar to morphine.
- It is used in morphine withdrawal, because of:
  - Its slow and persistent nature of action.
  - It accumulates in tissue and plasma $t_{1/2}$ on chronic use is 24–36 hours, hence once daily dosing needed.
  - Its sedative and subjective effects are less intense.
  - It is incapable of giving a "kick", and abuse potential is rated much lower than morphine.
  - Its high oral : parenteral ratio (1 : 2), hence oral therapy suffices.
  - Its high potency and affinity for opioid receptors.
- Two types of therapy are in use:
  1. *Substitution therapy*: 1mg oral dose of methadone can substitute 4 mg of morphine.
  2. *Maintenance therapy*: High dose of methadone is given over long-term to produce higher degree of tolerance so that pleasurable effects of IV doses of morphine are not perceived (cross-tolerance). Moreover, withdrawal symptoms of methadone are very mild and gradual.

61. Why does levodopa become ineffective in drug-induced parkinsonism? Explain.

- This is due to the following actions:

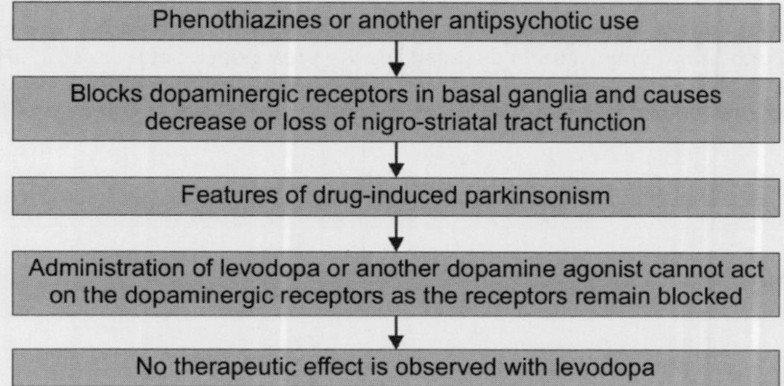

- Hence, in drug-induced parkinsonism, the mainstay of therapy is central anticholinergics or 1st generation antihistaminics (with anticholinergic side effects).

62. Carbidopa cannot be used as monotherapy in parkinsonism. Explain why?

- Carbidopa being an extracerebral decarboxylase inhibitor cannot penetrate the blood–brain barrier.
- Hence, if administered as monotherapy without in combination with levodopa, there would be no increased availability of dopamine is CNS, and thus, there would be no therapeutic benefit in parkinsonism.
- Only when in combination with levodopa, it increases dopamine availability in basal ganglia by decreasing peripheral conversion of levodopa to dopamine.

63. Why are levodopa and carbidopa combined in antiparkinsonian therapy? Explain.

- Carbidopa being an extracerebral decarboxylase inhibitor reduces peripheral conversion of levodopa to dopamine, and hence, increases the availability of dopamine in CNS, which is the therapeutic goal.
- The benefits of this combination are:
  - Plasma $t_{1/2}$ of levodopa is prolonged, and its dose is reduced to approximately ¼ th.
  - Systemic concentration of dopamine is reduced, so side effects are less prominent.
  - Therapeutic doses of dopamine in CNS are attained quickly.
  - Cardiac complications are minimized.
  - Pyridoxine reversal of dopa effect does not occur.
  - ON/OFF effect is minimized.
  - Degree of improvement may be higher.

64. Explain mechanism of action of tricyclic antidepressants (TCAs).

- The action is as follows:

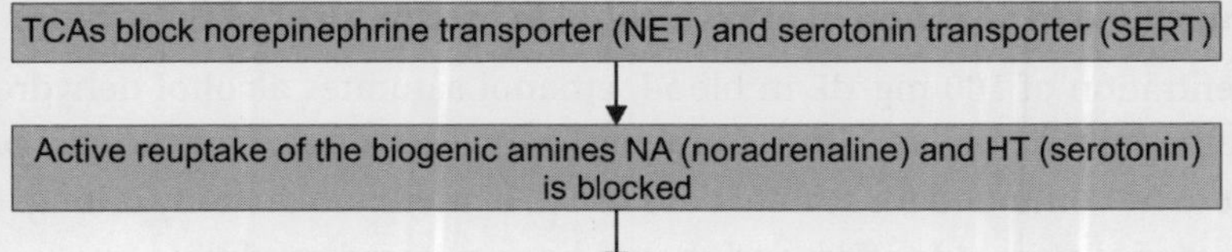

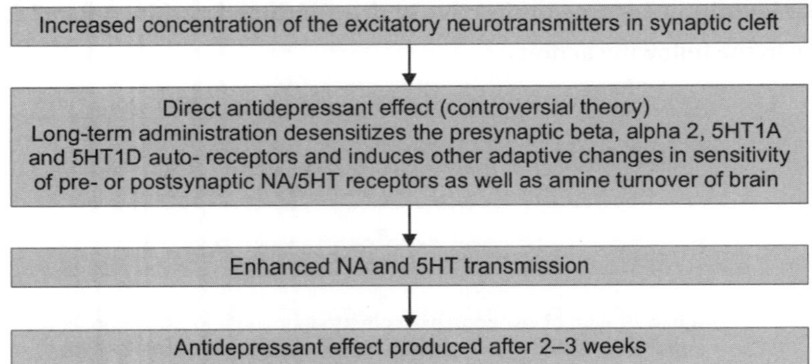

- Pharmacological actions:
  - *CNS*:
    - *On normals*:
      - Tiredness
      - Sleepiness
      - Unsteady gait
      - Provocation of anxiety
      - No euphoria or mood elevation.
    - *On depressed patients*:
      - Gradual mood elevation
      - Lower seizure threshold
      - *EEG*: Low dose produces hypnotic pattern; high dose causes desynchronization.
      - No euphoria.
    - Uptake blockade seems to initiate a series of time-dependent changes that culminate in the antidepressant effect.
  - *ANS*:
    - Potent anticholinergics—dry mouth, blurring of vision, constipation, urinary retention
    - Weak alpha 1 blocking action.
  - *CVS*:
    - Tachycardia
    - Postural hypotension
    - Cardiac arrhythmia
    - *ECG*: T wave inversion/suppression (most consistent change).

65. Explain mechanism of action of ethyl alcohol in methyl alcohol poisoning.

- At a concentration of 100 mg/dL in blood, ethanol saturates alcohol dehydrogenase and retards methanol metabolism. Thus, reducing formaldehyde and formic acid production.
- Treatment to be continued for several days as $T_{1/2}$ of methanol in body is long.
- However, ethanol gives side effect and should be monitored carefully.

66. Explain mechanism of action of dantrolene in malignant hyperthermia.

- Malignant hyperthermia is a genetically determined reaction which may be triggered by halothane (idiosyncrasy).
  - Subjects have an abnormal R_yR_1 receptor which when triggered leads to increased Ca^{2+} intracellularly- persistent muscle contraction → increased heat production.
  - Dantrolene selectively block R_yR_1 receptors and prevents Ca^{2+} induced Ca^{2+} release.

67. Explain mechanism of action of fluoxetine in depression.

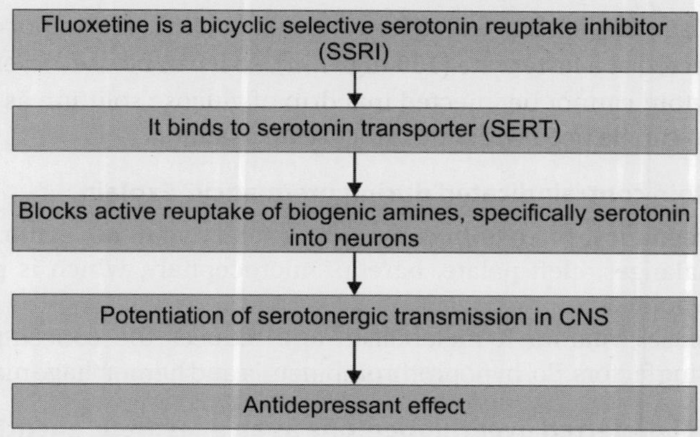

68. Why are centrally acting anticholinergics used in drug-induced parkinsonism? Explain.

- Centrally acting anticholinergics like trihexyphenidyl, biperiden, etc. are treatment of choice in drug-induced parkinsonism.
- Levodopa is not effective in this case, because:
  - Dopamine receptors are blocked.
  - There is no deficiency of dopamine.
    - Centrally acting anticholinergics have a higher central-peripheral anticholinergic action.
    - They act by reducing unbalanced cholinergic activity in the striatum brain in case of parkinsonism.
    - They are cheap and better tolerated. So, they are used in drug-induced parkinsonism.

69. Explain mechanism of action of valproate used as an antiepileptics.

- Valproic acid is a branched-chain aliphatic carboxylic acid with a broad-spectrum of anticonvulsant action.
- Valproate appears to exert its antiepileptic action via the following mechanism:
  - A phenytoin like frequency dependent prolongation of sodium channel inactivation
  - Weak attenuation of calcium-mediated T current like ethosuximide
  - Augmentation of release of inhibitory transmitters like GABA by inhibiting its degradation (by GABA transaminase) as well as by increasing its synthesis from glutamic acid.
- *Indications*:
  - 1st-line choice for:
    - Absence seizures

- Myoclonic seizures
- Atonic seizures
- Complex partial seizures
- 2nd-line choice for: GTCS.

70. Why is fosphenytoin preferred over phenytoin? Explain.

- Fosphenytoin is a water-soluble prodrug of phenytoin which has been introduced to overcome difficulties in IV administration of phenytoin.
- It is preferred over phenytoin because:
  - On IV administration, it is less damaging to vascular intima, only minor complications occur.
  - It can be injected at a faster rate (150 mg/min), so it can be used in emergency.
  - While phenytoin cannot be injected in a drip of glucose solution as it gets precipitated, fosphenytoin can be used with both glucose and saline.

71. Why is phenytoin contraindicated during pregnancy? Explain.

- Used during pregnancy, phenytoin can produce fetal hydantoin syndrome, manifested as hypoplastic phalanges, cleft palate, harelip, microcephaly, which is probably caused by arenoxide metabolite.
- Phenytoin increases vitamin K metabolism and reduces the concentration of vitamin K dependent clotting factors. So, hypoprothrombinemia and hemorrhage may occur in newborn.

72. Why is propofol preferred over thiopentone as an anesthetic agent? Explain.

- Propofol is an IV anesthetic, both for induction and as well as maintenance. It is particularly suited for the outpatient and surgery as:
  - Unconsciousness after propofol injection occurs in 15–45 seconds and lasts 5–10 minutes; elimination half-life is short (about 100 minutes). Its residual impairment is less marked and short lasting.
  - Incidence of postoperative nausea, vomiting is low, so patient compliance is very good.
- *Advantages over thiopentone:*
  - Elimination half-life is much shorter than thiopentone. This is due to rapid metabolism as thiopentone is stored in fatty tissues.
  - Laryngospasm may occur with thiopentone, but propofol lacks airway irritation.
  - Residual impairment is more marked in thiopentone.

73. Explain mechanism of action of alprazolam used as hypnotic.

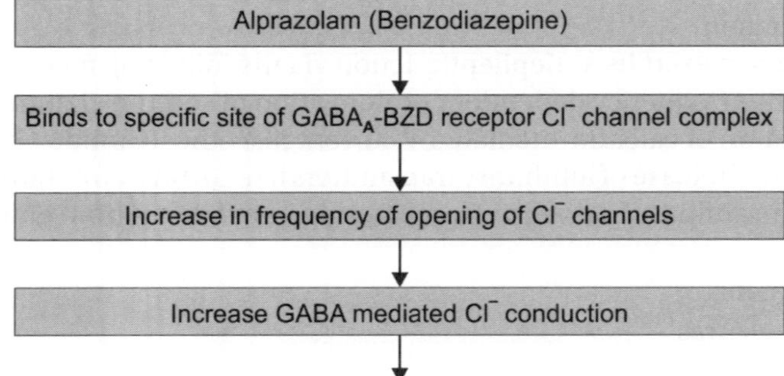

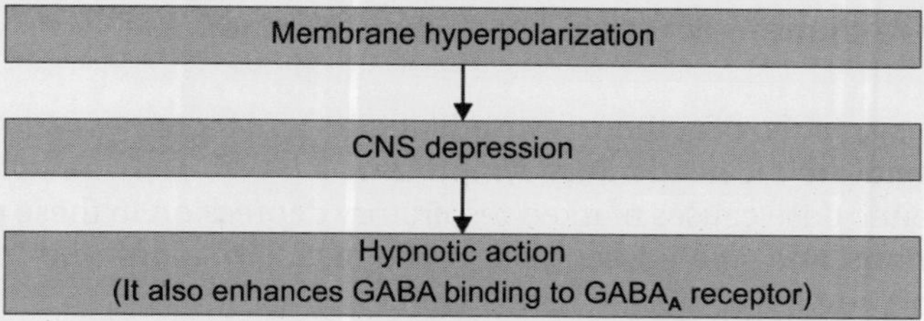

74. Why is levodopa reserved for severe cases of parkinsonism? Explain.

- Levodopa is the drug of choice for idiopathic parkinsonism, but it is reserved for severe cases only, because:
  - Oxidative metabolism of dopamine leads to increased reactive oxygen species (ROS), thus causing neural degeneration. According to this theory, levodopa may provide symptomatic relief but accelerate disease progression.
  - Appearance of dyskinesia is related to dose and duration of levodopa therapy.
- So, for mild disease therapy is initiated with anticholinergics, selegiline or newer DA agonist like ropinirole, pramipexole or amantadine.

75. Explain mechanism of action of lithium in bipolar disorder.

Lithium in therapeutic concentration inhibits hydrolysis of inositol-1-phosphate by inositol monophosphatase leads to supply of free inositol for production of IP_3 and DAG is reduced → selectively dampen signal transduction in overactive receptor functioning through PI_3 hydrolysis → desired effect on bipolar disorder due to membrane stabilization crystal.

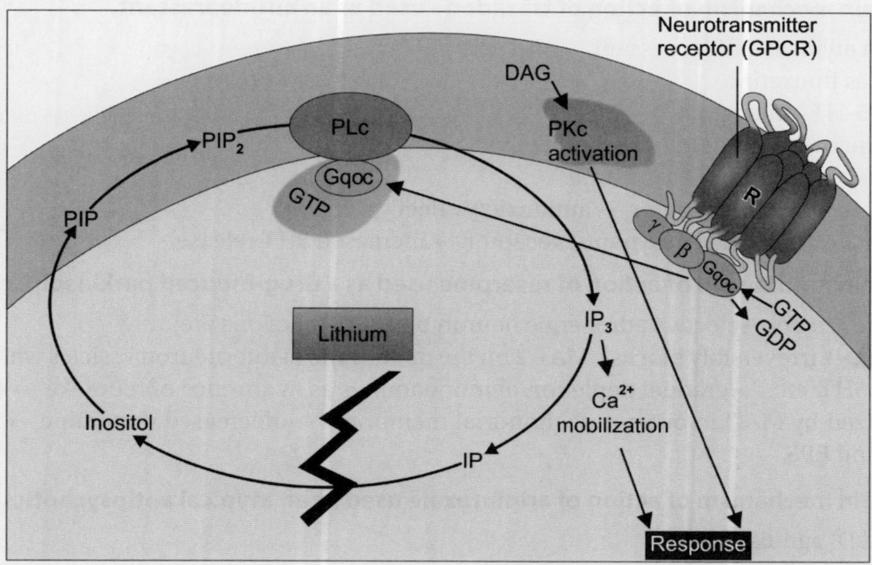

Fig. 6.5: MOA of lithium at cellular level

76. Why is morphine contraindicated in head injury? Explain.

- This is because:
  - By retaining carbon dioxide, there is vasodilatation and increase in intracranial pressure, which will aggravate the head injury symptoms.
  - Even therapeutic dose causes marked respiratory depression in these patients.
  - Vomiting, miosis and altered sensorium produced by morphine interferes with the assessment of progress of disease in head injury cases.

77. Why are SSRI preferred over TCA for treatment of depression? Explain.

- TCAs are 1st-generation antidepressants while SSRIs are of 2nd generation.
- Causes of preference of SSRIs are twofold:
  - Disadvantages of TCAs:
    - Frequent anticholinergic, CVS and neurological side effects
    - Relatively lower safety margin
    - Fatalities common in overdose
    - Lag time of 2–4 weeks before antidepressant effect manifests
    - Significant number of patients respond incompletely and some do not.
  - Advantages of SSRIs:
    - Produce little or no sedation
    - Do not interfere with cognitive/psychomotor function
    - Do not have anticholinergic side effects
    - Devoid of alpha adrenergic blocking action—suitable for elderly patients as there is no postural hypotension
    - Practically no seizure precipitating propensity
    - Does not inhibit cardiac conduction, hence in overdose, life threatening arrhythmias are not a problem.

78. Explain mechanism of action of trazadone used as an antidepressant.

- It is an atypical antidepressant.
- Same as fluoxetine
- Weak 5-HT_2 antagonist
- Prominent α_1 adrenergic blocker
- Decreased reuptake of serotonin
- Blockade of $5HT_{1A}$ receptor → antianxiety effect
- Desensitization 5HT presynaptic receptor → increased 5HT release.

79. Explain mechanism of action of reserpine used as a drug-induced parkinsonism.

Reserpine is a non-selective adrenergic neuron blocker. Its actions are:
Reserpine → irreversibly blocks VMAT-2 on the membrane of interneuron vesicles which store NA, DA, 5HT, etc. → gradual depletion of monoamines as in absence of reuptake → they are metabolized by MAO in outer mitochondrial membrane → decreased dopamine → parkinsonism and EPS.

80. Explain mechanism of action of aripiprazole used as an atypical antipsychotics.

- Partial D_2 agonist
- 5HT1A agonist
- 5HT2A antagonist

CARDIOVASCULAR DRUGS

81. Explain mechanism of action of thiazide diuretics used in hypertension.

- Initially the diuretics reduce plasma and ECF volume by 5–15% and this reduces cardiac output → blood pressure decreases.

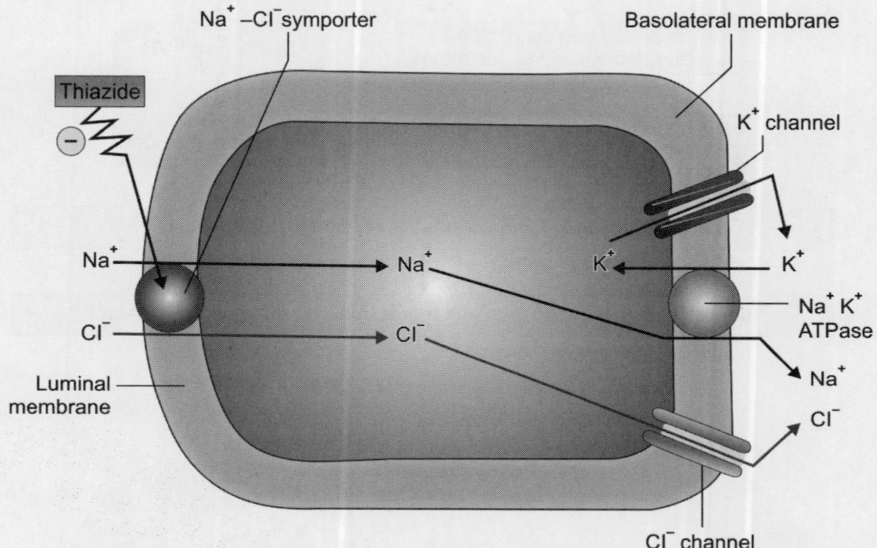

Fig. 6.6: MOA of thiazide at cellular level

- Inhibits NaCl transport in the early segment of DCT → natriuresis → decreased preload by renal effects → decreased cardiac output → decreased blood pressure.
- Slow decrease of total peripheral resistance (raised initially) during chronic treatment.
- Small persisting Na^+ and volume deficit → decreased Na^+ concentration in vascular smooth muscle → reduces stiffness of vessel wall and dampens responsiveness to constrictor stimuli (noradrenaline, angiotensin II).
- A mild slowly developing vasodilator action of thiazide due to opening of smooth muscle ATP sensitive K^+ channel and hyperpolarization.

82. Why is nitroglycerin (IV) the drug of choice in LVF? Explain.

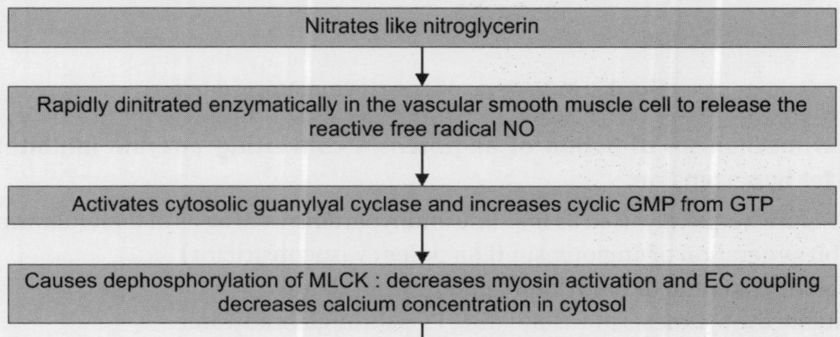

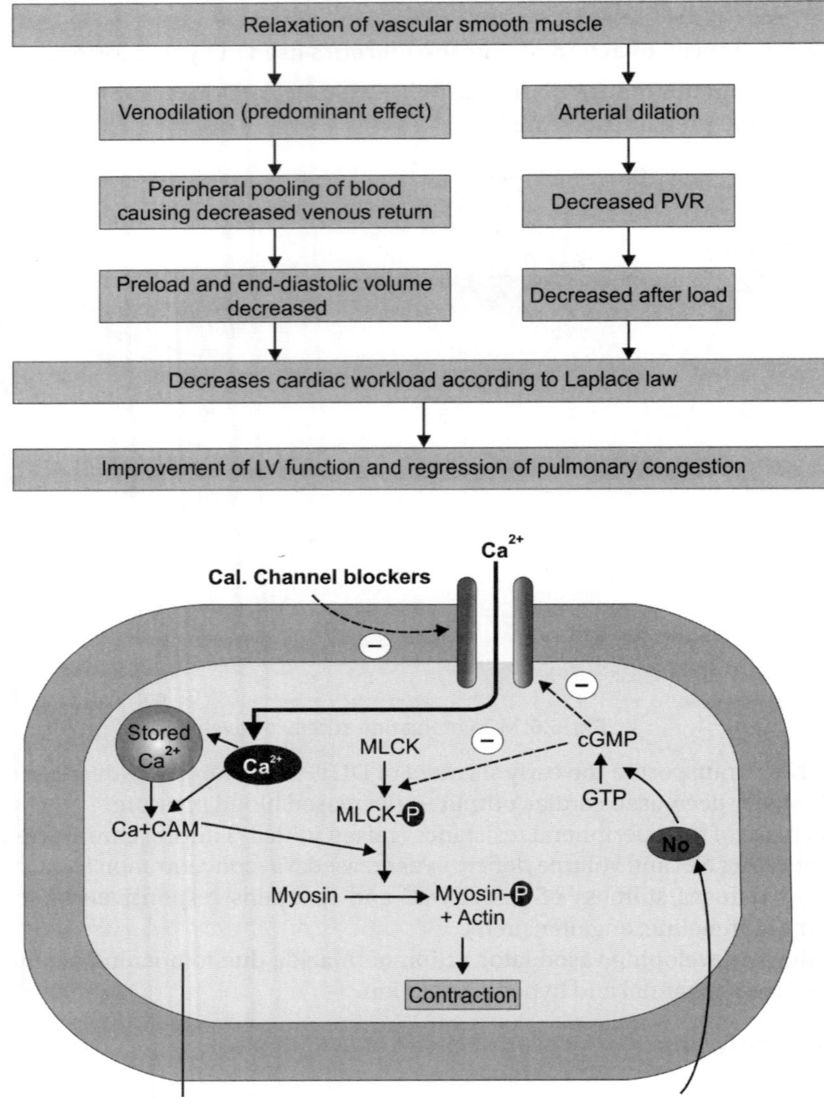

Fig. 6.7: MOA of various negative inotropic drugs

83. Explain mechanism of action of angiotensin converting enzyme inhibitors (ACEIs) indicated for hypertension.

- The ACEIs are frequently used as first-line antihypertensive drug as of their following actions:
  - Inhibit generation of angiotensin II (a potent vasoconstrictor)
  - Inhibit degradation of bradykinin, potent vasodilator
  - Stimulate the synthesis of vasodilating PGs through bradykinin
  - Reduce sympathetic system activity.

84. Why is sildenafil contraindicated with nitrate? Explain.

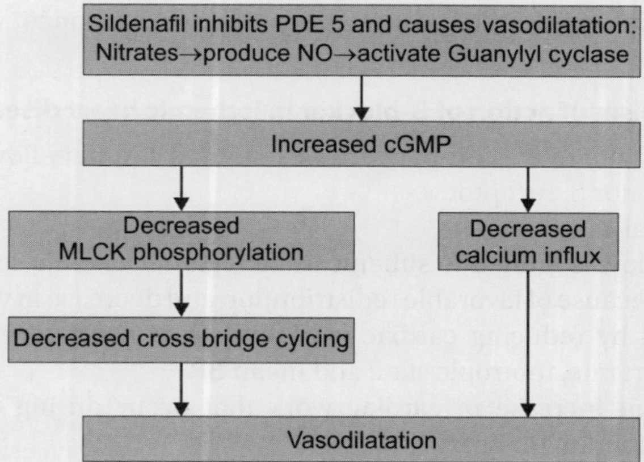

- Moreover, sildenafil also increases cyclic-GMP and thus ultimately coadministration leads to dangerous vasodilatation and hypotensive crisis.

85. Explain mechanism of action of morphine in LVF.

- In cases of LVF, morphine IV infusion affords dramatic relief by:
  - Reducing preload on heart due to vasodilation and peripheral pooling of blood
  - Tendency to shift blood from pulmonary to systemic circuit thus relieves pulmonary congestion and edema
  - Allays air hunger and dyspnea by depressing respiratory center
  - Cuts down sympathetic stimulation by calming the patient, thereby reducing cardiac workload.

86. Explain mechanism of action of dopamine in CHF.

- Dopamine (at a concentration of <2 μg/kg/min) → acts on D_1 receptor → dilates renal, coronary and mesenteric blood vessels → increased GFR and urine output.
- Dopamine (at a concentration of 2–10 μg/kg/min) → stimulates β_1 receptor → increased myocardial contractility and cardiac output.
- CHF → ventricles dilated and unable to develop sufficient wall tension → decreased ejaculation of blood → increased pressure on pulmonary trunk → increased backward pressure on IVC and SVC and leads to development of pulmonary edema.
- Thus, dopamine by increasing cardiac contractility and urine output helps in treatment of CHF.

87. Explain mechanism of action of digoxin used in heart failure.

- Na^+–K^+ATPase is a membrane bound enzyme which is called digitalis receptor.
- It is also called sodium pump.
- Digitalis → binds and inhibits Na^+–K^+ATPase → increases intracellular Na^+ → decreased extrusion of Ca^{2+} via $3Na^+$–$1Ca^{2+}$ exchanger, entry of Ca^{2+} into cardiac cell via L-type Ca^{2+} channel during action potential and vCa^{2+} induced Ca^{2+} influx from endoplasmic reticulum via RYR2 → increased Ca^{2+} uptake and storage in sarcoplasmic reticulum → increased amount of Ca^{2+} released from SR during each action potential → increased availability of

Ca^{2+} for excitation–contraction coupling → thus increasing myocardial contractility (+ve inotropic effect) → increased cardiac output.

[Digoxin increases myocardial contractility and performance without increasing O_2 demand].

88. Explain mechanism of action of β-blocker in ischemic heart disease.

- Beta-blocker does not dilate coronary arteries → total coronary flow is rather reduced due to blockade of dilator β_2 receptor.
- They are beneficial as:
  - Reduction of flow is limited to subepicardial region, ischemic subendocardial region is not reduced, because of favorable redistribution and decrease in ventricular wall tension.
  - β-blockers act by reducing cardiac work and O_2 consumption as a consequence of decreased heart rate, inotropic state and mean BP.
  - β-blockers limit increase in cardiac work that occur during exercise or anxiety by antiadrenergic action on heart.
  - β-blockers prevent arrhythmia.

89. Explain mechanism of action of Na^+-nitroprusside in hypertensive emergency.

- Sodium nitroprusside is a rapidly (within seconds) and consistently acting vasodilator and has brief duration of action (2–5 minutes) so that vascular tone can be titrated with the rate of IV infusion.
- So, it is popular in treatment of hypertensive emergency and both as venodilator and arteriodilator.

90. Explain mechanism of action of digoxin in atrial fibrillation.

- It is used for controlling ventricular rate in AF whether associated with CHF or not. Digoxin reduces the ventricular rate in AF by decreasing no of impulses that are able to pass down the AV node and bundle of His.
  - It increases ERP of AV node by direct vagomimetic effect and antiadrenergic action. The minimal interval between two consecutive impulses that can successfully traverse the conducting tissue, increases.
  - Because of relatively long ERP of AV node, many of atrial impulses falling in relative refractory period get extinguished by this type of conduction. These concealed impulses nevertheless leave the upper margin of AV node refractory for a further period. Digoxin increases the number of concealed impulses and indirectly prolongs the interval between any two impulses that are successfully conducted to ventricle.
- When digoxin is given in atrial fibrillation, average ventricular rate decreases in a dose dependent manner and pulse deficit is abolished. It is particularly effective in ventricular rate at rest.

91. Explain mechanism of action of lignocaine used in arrhythmia.

- Lignocaine is a popular antiarrhythmic in intensive care unit.
- The mechanism of action is:
  - Lignocaine is a blocker of Na^+ channel more than open state, such as it is relatively selective for partially depolarized cells and these with longer APD (where Na^+ channels remain inactivated for a longer time).

- The most prominent cardiac action is suppression of automaticity in ectopic foci. Enhanced phase-4 depolarization in partially depolarized or stretched PFs and after depolarization are antagonized, but SA node automaticity is not depressed.
- Enhances K^+ efflux in phase-3 and shortens duration of ventricular action potential.
- ERP is reduced, hence ERP/APD ratio is increased.
- Reduces anatomical reentry by either removing one-way block or producing two-way block.

92. Explain mechanism of action of morphine in AMI.

- Morphine being a potent opioid analgesic relieves pain, apprehension, anxiety in a patient of AMI by acting on μ receptor.
- Morphine's analgesic property has both spinal and supraspinal components, hence relieves diffuse and dull visceral pain better.
- Morphine causes vasodilation by:
  - Histamine release
  - Depression of vasomotor center
  - Direct decreasing tone of blood vessels
  - Vasodilation—decreased PVR—decreased cardiac load—antiischemic property
- Increase ventricular fibrillation threshold which is a complication of AMI.

93. Why is furosemide the drug of choice in acute pulmonary edema? Explain.

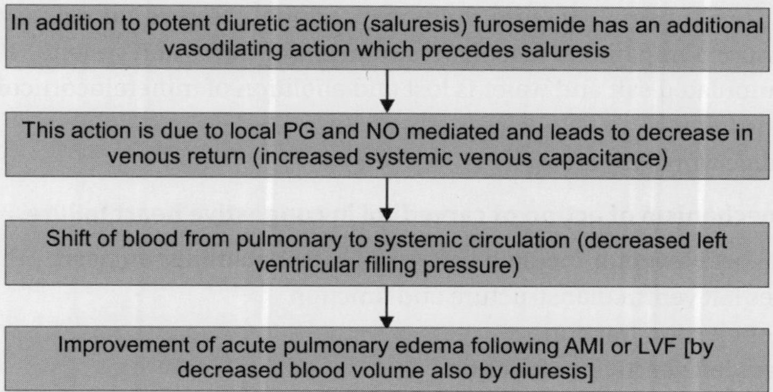

94. Explain mechanism of action of β-blocker used as an antihypertensive.

- Block β-1→ negative inotropic and chronotropic → decreased contractility and heart rate → BP falls.
- 3rd-generation β-blockers have additional α-blocking action → decreased BP due to vasodilation.
- Decreased Na^+ release from sympathetic terminals due to blockade of β mediated facilitation of release process.
- β_1 mediated renin release from kidney decreased → decreased Na^+ and H_2O retention → BP falls.
- Weak central action, reducing central sympathetic outflow, since poorly cross blood brain barrier.

95. Explain mechanism of action of β-blockers in heart failure.

- β-blockers are useful in mild-to-moderate heart failure.
- Long-term therapy with these beta-blockers improve symptoms.
  - Immediate hemodynamic action of beta-blockers is to depress cardiac contractility and ejection fraction; these parameters gradually improve over time. After couple of months, ejection fraction is gradually higher than baseline.
  - Beta-blockers antagonize sympathetic overactivity in CHF and thus antagonize ventricular wall stress enhancing, apoptosis promoting and pathological remodeling effect.
  - Beta-blockers lower plasma markers of sympathetic, RAS and endothelin.

96. Explain mechanism of action of ACEI in heart failure.

- ACE inhibitors afford symptomatic as well as disease modifying benefits in CCF.
  - Inhibit generation of angiotensin II, a potent vasoconstrictor.
  - Inhibit degradation of bradykinin, a potent vasodilator.
  - Stimulate generation of vasodilating PGs and nitric oxide.
  - Reduce sympathetic nervous system activity.
  - Retard ventricular hypertrophy, myocardial cell apoptosis, fibrosis, intracellular matrix change and remodeling. Thus, they:
    - Reduce both preload and afterload.
    - Reduce right atrial pressure, pulmonary arterial pressure, pulmonary capillary wedge pressure, sympathetic vascular resistance, wall stress and systemic BP.
    - Accumulated salt and water is lost and abolition of mineralocorticoid mediated Na^+ retention.
    - Cardiac work is decreased.

97. Explain mechanism of action of carvedilol in congestive heart failure.

- Blockage of beta receptor mediated effects of catecholamines on heart
  - Improves left ventricular structure and function
  - Increases ejection fraction
  - Decreases left ventricular function
  - Decreases promotion of apoptosis.
- Prevention of sinister arrhythmia
- Lowers plasma markers of activation of sympathetic, RAS and endothelin-1
- Has antioxidant effect.

98. Explain mechanism of action of dopamine in cardiogenic shock.

- Dopamine, a sympathomimetic agent, increases blood pressure by acting on vascular α_1 receptor
- Improves circulation, and has positive inotropic, chronotropic, dromotropic, bathmotropic via β_1 stimulation
- Selectively dilates renal, mesenteric and coronary blood vessels by acting on D_1 receptor and improves blood supply to vital organs.

99. Why is propranolol contraindicated in variant angina? Explain.

Pathogenesis of variant angina—attacks are unpredictable and caused by recurrent coronary vasospasm:

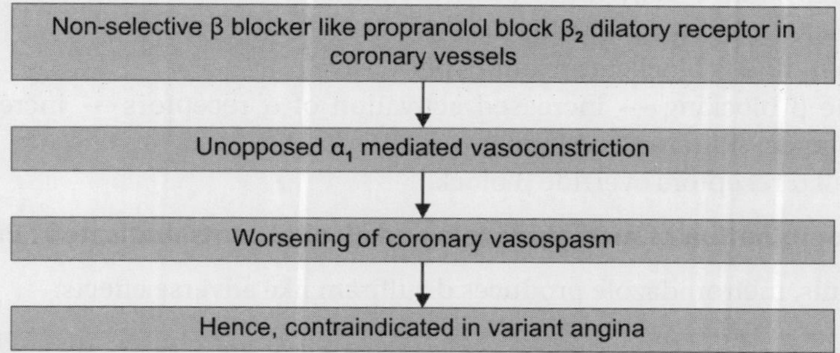

100. Abrupt clonidine withdrawal is not done. Explain why?

- Clonidine acts as follows:

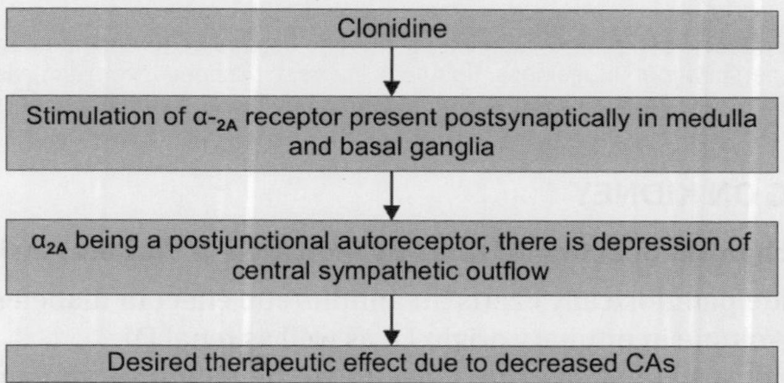

- Abrupt clonidine withdrawal results in anxiety, alarming rise in BP, tachycardia, restlessness, sweating, headache, nausea and vomiting.
- This is because:
  - Sudden removal of inhibition of central sympathetic outflow resulting in release of large amount of stored CAs.
  - Supersensitivity of peripheral adrenergic receptors to CAs that develop due to chronic reduction of sympathetic tone, i.e. receptor upregulation.
  - This is similar to that of pheochromocytoma.

101. Both α- and β-blockers are used in pheochromocytoma. Explain why?

- Tumors of adrenal medullary cells → excess catecholamines → intermittent/persistent hypertension.
  - *Use of α-blocker*:
    - Due to excess catecholamines blood volume is low (due to shift from vascular to extravascular space). Treatment with α-blocker normalize blood volume and distribution of body water.
    - Pouring of CAs in blood during surgery → marked rise of blood pressure. Use of α-blocker in pre-, post- and intraoperatively.

  - Removal of tumor → marked fall in BP due to vessel dilation. α-blockers restore blood volume if administered before.
- *Use of β-blocker*:
  - Used to control tachycardia and arrhythmia.
  - Reduce cardiomyopathy due to CA.
  - Both α- and β-blockers are antihypertensive.
  - Alone β blocking → increased activation of α receptors → increased peripheral resistance → increased blood pressure
- Activation of α receptors override β block.

102. Why is combination of metronidazole and alcohol contraindicated? Explain.

In some patients, metronidazole produces disulfiram like adverse effects:

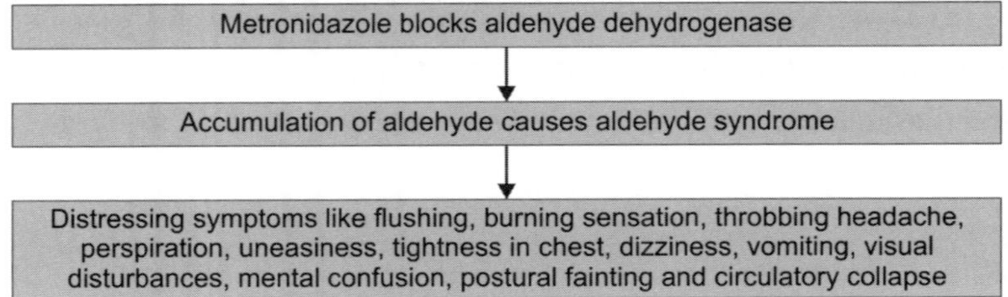

DRUGS ACTING ON KIDNEY

103. Explain mechanism of action of thiazide indicated in diabetes insipidus (DI).

- Diuretic thiazide paradoxically exerts an antidiuretic effect in diabetes insipidus. Thiazide reduces urine volume in pituitary origin DI as well as renal DI.
- Thiazide induces a state of sustained electrolyte depletion → glomerular filtrate is more completely reabsorbed iso-osmotically → further reduced salt reabsorption in cortical diluting segment → a smaller volume of less dilute urine is presented and same is passed out.
- Secondly, thiazides reduce GFR and thus fluid load on tubules.

104. Explain mechanism of action of tolvaptan as antidiuretics.

- It is an orally active nonpeptide selective V_2 receptor antagonist which is used for treatment of hyponatremia due to CHF, cirrhosis of liver and SIADH.
- It increases free water clearance by kidney and helps correct low plasma Na^+ level.

105. Atracurium is safe in patients with renal impairment. Explain how.

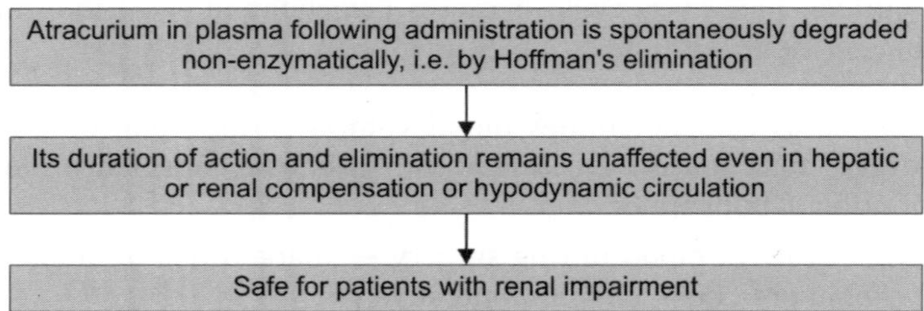

106. Explain mechanism of action of erythropoietin indicated for chronic renal failure-induced anemia.

- EPO is a sialoglycoprotein hormone encoded by a single copy gene of chromosome 7 that is expressed primarily in peritubular interstitial cells of kidney.
- It is one of the erythropoiesis-stimulating agents (ESA) in our body, the release of which is stimulated by anemia or hypoxemia sensed by kidney cells and synthesis rapidly increases by 100-fold or more.

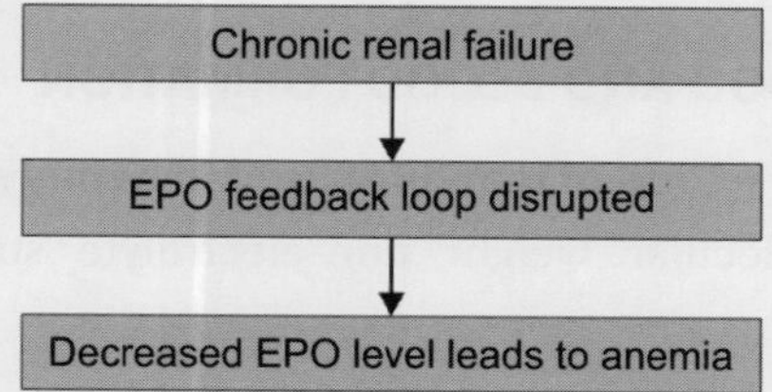

- On administration of EPO by IV or SC injection, it corrects anemia by the following mechanism of action:
  - Stimulates erythropoiesis from BFU-E/ CFU-E onward and enhances their maturation to RBCs
  - Stimulates proliferation of BFU-E/ CFU-E cells
  - Induces Hb formation
  - Releases reticulocytes in the circulation.
- Signal transduction at molecular level:
  - EPO binds to specific receptors on its target cells which are JAK-STAT binding receptors that alter phosphorylation of intracellular proteins and activate transcription factors to regulate specific gene expression.
  - EPO induces erythropoiesis on dose-dependent manner but has no effect on RBC life span.

107. Explain mechanism of action of α-calcidiol used in chronic renal failure.

- Normal process of vitamin D activation:

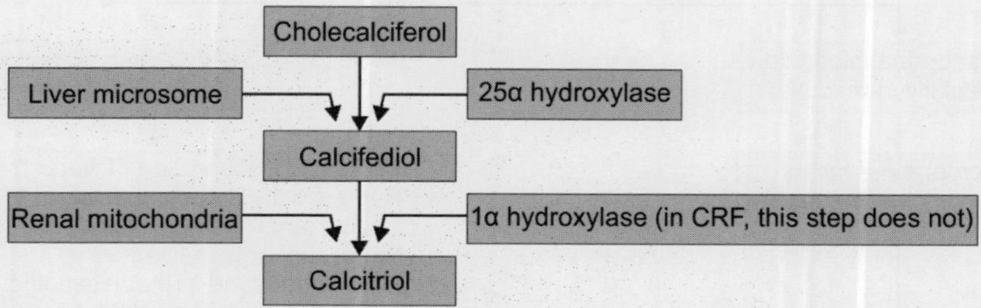

- In CRF, 1α hydroxylase is inhibited due to low level.
- α-calcidiol directly metabolized to calcitriol in liver, hence vitamin D_3 level are retained and Ca^{2+} is normal.

108. Explain mechanism of action of enalapril used in diabetic nephropathy.

- Prolonged ACEI therapy has been found to prevent or delay end-stage renal disease in type 1 as well as type 2 DM.

- Albuminemia (an index of glomerulopathy) remains stable in these treated with ACEI.
- Increased creatinine clearance requires less dialysis and longer life expectancy.
- Above benefits are due to the following mechanism of action:
  - Systemic and intrarenal hemodynamic change
  - Decreased abnormal mesangial cell growth
  - Decreased interglomerular pressure and hyperfiltration
  - Oragn protective role due to decreased micro- and macrovascular complications of DM.

DRUGS AFFECTING BLOOD AND BLOOD FORMATION

109. Explain mechanism of action of mannitol used in hemolytic reaction.

- Mannitol is a low-molecular weight non-electrolyte substance which is pharmacodynamically inert.

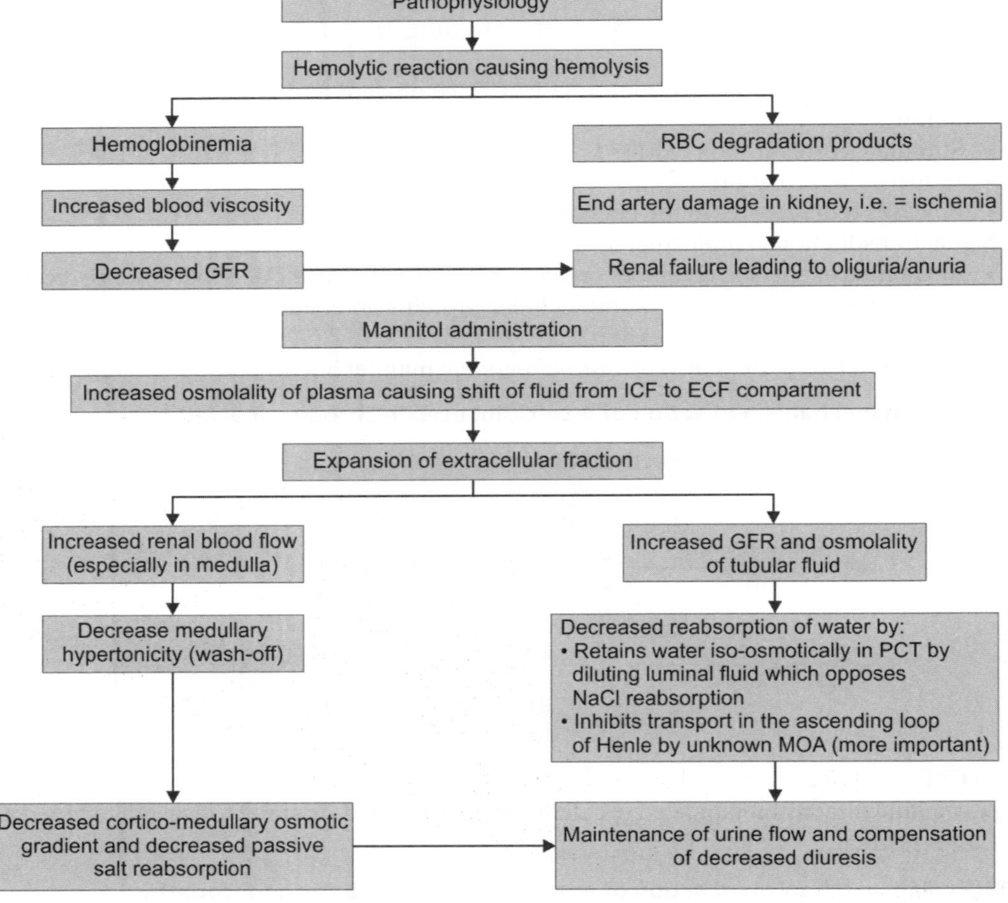

- However, mannitol is contraindicated if acute kidney injury sets in.

110. Low-molecular-weight heparin (LMWH) administration does not need laboratory monitoring. Explain why?

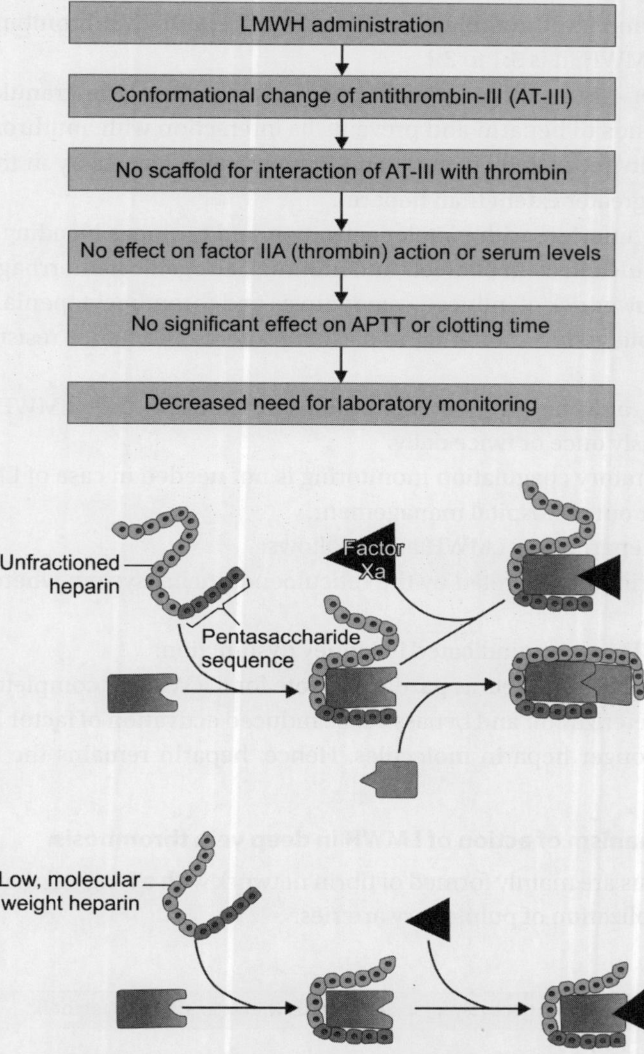

Fig. 6.8: Mechanism of action of heparin and LMWH

111. LMWH is preferred over unfractionated heparin but unfractionated heparin has some advantages too. Explain why?

- Both unfractionated heparin and LMWH have no intrinsic anticoagulant activity. Instead these agents bind to antithrombin and accelerates the rate at which it inhibits various coagulation proteases.

- Advantages of LMWH over heparin are as follows:
  - Both heparin and LMWH bind to antithrombin via a specific pentasaccharide sequence but all molecules of LMWH do not possess enough saccharide units to cause bridging of thrombin and antithrombin. Thus, in case of heparin, Xa:thrombin inhibition is 1:1, whereas in LMWH, it is 3:1 to 2:1.
  - Platelet factor 4 is a cationic protein released from the alpha granules during platelet activation, binds to heparin and prevents its interaction with antithrombin. LMWH has a lower affinity for platelet factor 4 and hence retains its activity in the vicinity of such thrombi to a greater extent than heparin.
  - Heparin may interfere with platelet activation and prolongs bleeding time; in contrast, LMWH has little effect on platelets and minimal iatrogenic hemorrhagic complications.
  - LMWH has lower risk of induced osteoporosis and thrombocytopenia.
  - LMWH exhibits reduced binding to plasma proteins and hence resistance to LMWH is rare.
  - Heparin can only be given by continuous IV infusion, but LMWH is administered subcutaneously once or twice daily.
  - Routine laboratory coagulation monitoring is not needed in case of LMWH and may be used even for out of hospital management.
- Advantages of heparin over LMWH are as follows:
  - Heparin is primarily excreted by the reticuloendothelial system whereas LMWH by the kidneys.
  - Hence, LMWH is contraindicated in kidney dysfunction.
  - Protamine sulfate only acts as partial antidote for LMWH but complete for heparin.
  - Cardiac catheterization and bypass cause induced activation of factor XII which is better blocked by longer heparin molecules. Hence, heparin remains the drug of choice in these cases.

112. Explain mechanism of action of LMWH in deep vein thrombosis.

- Venous thrombus are mainly formed of fibrin network with a long tail that can easily detach and cause embolization of pulmonary arteries.

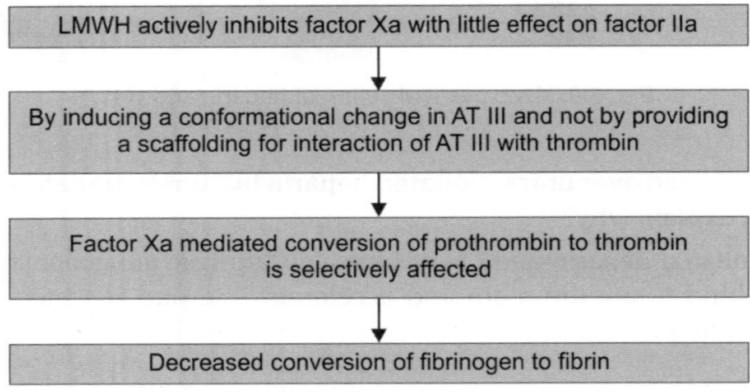

113. Vitamin B_{12} and folic acid are coadministered in megaloblastic anemia. Explain why?

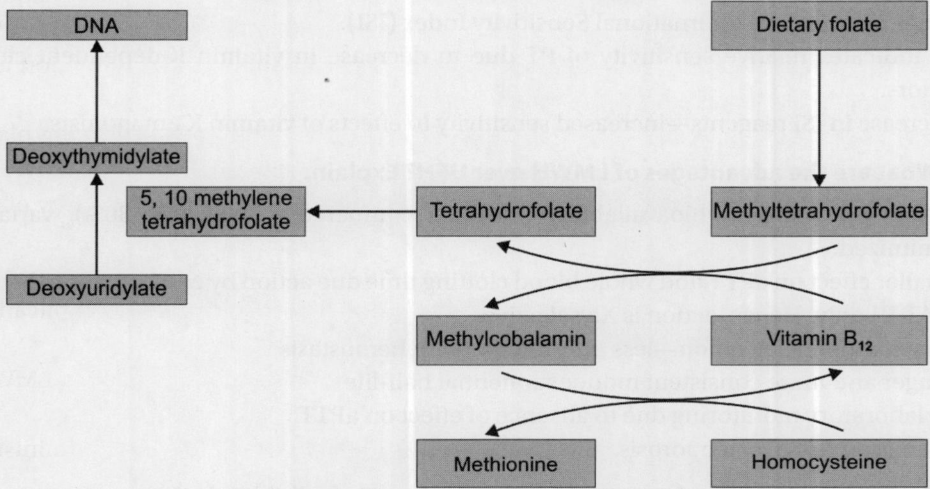

Fig. 6.9: Interrelated role of vit. B12 and folice acid in DNA synthesis

- In case of only folic acid deficiency, there is decreased methyl THFA and hence retarded DNA synthesis.
- In case of only vitamin B_{12} deficiency, there is trapping of folate as methyl THFA in the absence of THF (folate trap hypothesis).
- Hence, it is clear that both are required in adequate amounts for normal DNA synthesis and hence used in combination in megaloblastic anemia.
- In case of folic acid monotherapy, neurological symptoms increase due to demyelination causing subacute combined degeneration of spinal cord. Vitamin B_{12} is thus essential along with it.

114. Why has warfarin a delayed onset of action? Explain

- Warfarin exerts anticoagulant effect by decreased gamma-carboxylation of glutamate residues of vitamik K- dependent factors II, VII, IX and X.
- Plasma half-lives of these are:
  - Factor VII : 6 hours
  - Factor IX : 24 hours
  - Factor X : 40 hours
  - Prothrombin (factor II) : 60 hours
- Though syntheses of the clotting factors diminish within 2–4 hours of warfarin administration, anticoagulant effect develops gradually over next 103 days. Levels of clotting factors already present in plasma gradually decline during this period. Even larger initial doses hasten the effect only slightly as there is no effect on already synthesized factors.

115. Why are oral anticoagulants needed to be individualized? Explain.

- Prothrombin time (PT) varies in individuals

- PT is prolonged when functional levels of fibrinogen, factor V or vitamin K-dependent clotting factors II, VII, IX, and X are decreased.
- Drugs have variant International Sensitivity Index (ISI).
- ISI indicates relative sensitivity of PT due to decrease in vitamin K-dependent clotting factors.
- Decrease in ISI reagents—increased sensitivity to effects of vitamin K antagonists.

116. What are the advantages of LMWH over UFH? Explain.

- Better subcutaneous bioavailability (70–90%) compared to UFH (20–30%), variability minimized.
- Smaller effect on aPTT and whole blood clotting time due action by conformational change of AT-III only. Hence, action is Xa selective.
- Lesser antiplatelet action—less interference with hemostasis
- Longer and more consistent monoexponential half-life
- No laboratory monitoring due to absence of effect on aPTT.
- Decreased risk of osteoporosis.

117. Explain mechanism of action of statins used as a hypolipidemic drugs.

- Statins are the most effective agents for treating hyperlipidemia.
- They act by:
  - Competitively inhibiting HMG-CoA reductase, the rate limiting step in cholesterol biosynthesis. Therapeutic dose decreases cholesterol by 20–50%.
  - This results in compensatory increase in LDL receptor expression on liver cells→ increased receptor mediated catabolism of IDL and LDL over long-term, feedback induction of HMG-CoA reductase with a dose dependent lowering of LDL cholesterol level.
  - They also increase HDL and decrease LDL.

118. Explain mechanism of action of clopidogrel used as an antiplatelet.

- Active metabolite of clopidogrel → alters surface receptor on platelets and inhibits ADP as well as fibrinogen-induced platelet aggregation.
- Active metabolite of clopidogrel → irreversibly blocks Gi coupled $P2Y_{12}$ type of purinergic receptor which mediate adenyl cyclase inhibition due to ADP → activation of platelet is interfered → antiplatelet effect.

119. Explain mechanism of action of aspirin used as an antithrombotics.

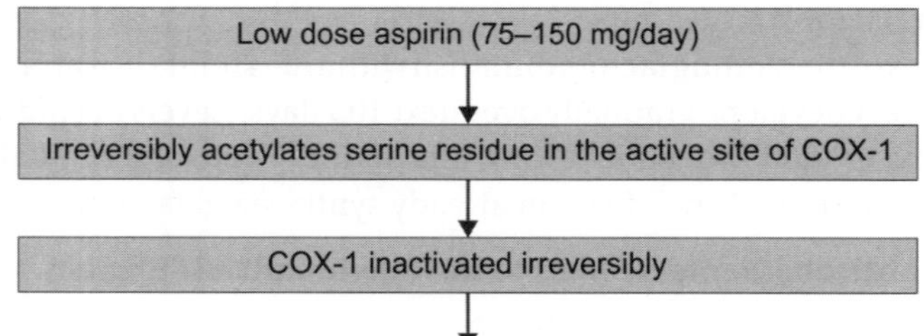

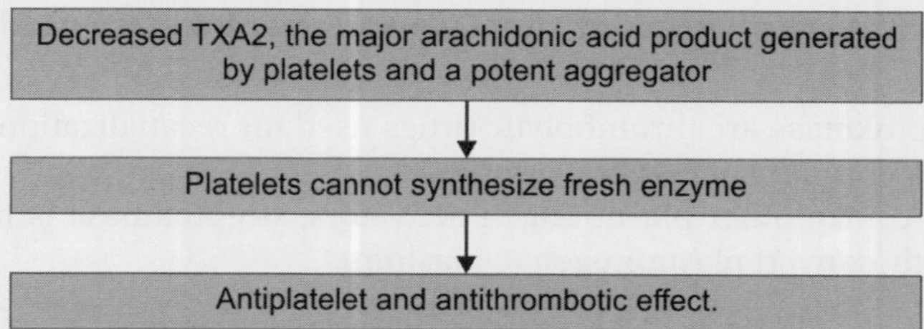

120. Explain mechanism of action of abciximab used as an antiplatelet.

Abciximab is the F_{ab} fragment of a chimeric monoclonal antibody against Gp IIb/IIIa protein.

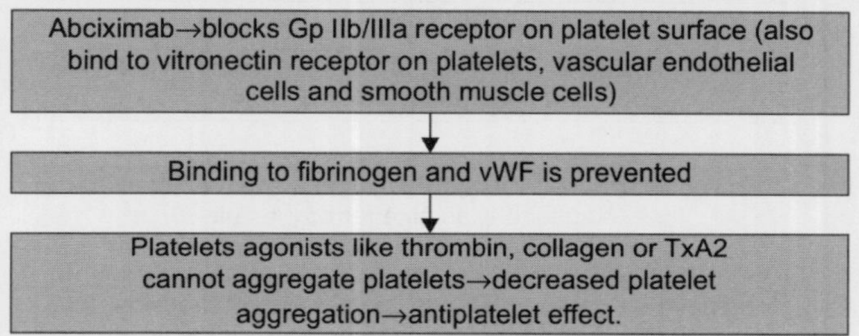

121. Explain mechanism of action of heparin used as an anticoagulant.

- Heparin binds to and activates antithrombin-III (serine proteinase inhibitor) → heparin AT-III binds to clotting factors of intrinsic and common pathway → factor Xa, IXa, Xia, XIIa are inhibited → anticoagulant effect.
- As low concemntration of heparin, factor Xa mediated conversion of prothombin to thrombin is selectively affected. The anticoagulant action is exerted mainly by inhibition of factor Xa as well as thrombin-mediated conversion of fibrinogen to fibrin.
- Heparin in high doses inhibits platelet aggregation.

122. Explain mechanism of action of warfarin used as ananticoagulant.

Warfarin is a coumarin derivative and has structural similarity to that of vitamin K.

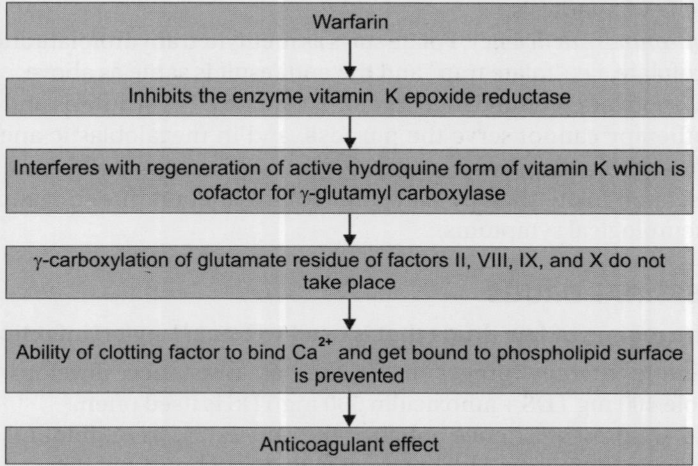

123. Explain mechanism of action of alteplase and streptokinase used as a thrombolytic agents.

- Alteplase/streptokinase are thrombolytic drugs used for recanalization of occluded blood vessels (usually coronary or cerebral arteries).
- *Streptokinase*: Unlike other plasminogen activators, streptokinase is not an enzyme and does not directly convert plasminogen to plasmin.

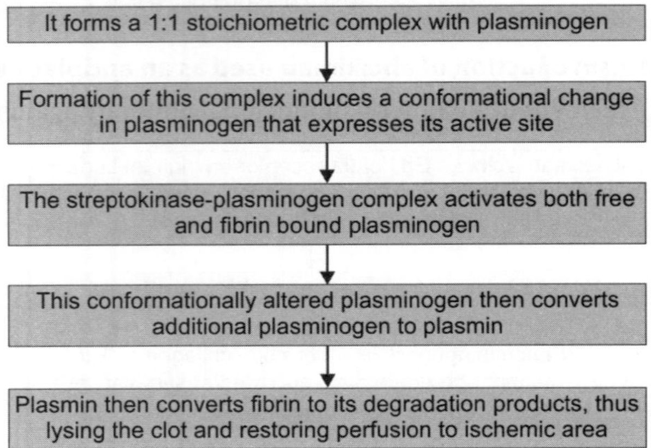

- *Alteplase*:
  - It is a recombinant tissue plasminogen activator.
  - It is moderately specific for fibrin bound plasminogen. Alteplase consists of five discrete domains of which interaction with fibrin is mediated by the finger domain and to a lesser extent by second kringle domain.
  - Rest of the mechanism is same as above.

124. Why are vitamin B_{12} and folic acid coadministered in megaloblastic anemia? Explain.

- The actions if vitamin B_{12} and folic acid are interrelated in DNA synthesis and cell division. Thus, isolated deficiency or deficiency of both causes nucleocytoplasmic asynchrony in marrow, and finally, megaloblastic anemia in peripheral blood smear.
  - *Isolated folic acid deficiency*: Decreased methyltetrahydrofolate, finally leading to decreased DNA synthesis.
  - *Isolated vitamin B_{12} deficiency*: Folate stays as methyltetrahydrofolate and is not converted tetrahydrofolate, i.e. "folate trap" and the end result is same as above.
- It is clear that both are required together for adequate DNA synthesis and RBC maturation. Thus, monotherapy cannot serve the purpose, and in megaloblastic anemia, always dual therapy is the treatment of choice.
- Moreover, isolated folate therapy may impede myelination due to vitamin B_{12} deficiency and cause neurological symptoms.

GASTROINTESTINAL DRUGS

125. Explain the regime of few drugs that is used to treat *H. pylori* infection.

- Single antibiotic therapy proves ineffective as resistance develops rapidly. Hence, metronidazole 400 mg TDS + amoxicillin 500 mg TDS is used often.
- PPIs are acid suppressors, hence enhance the anti-*H. pylori* antibiotics. Optimum effects are obtained if pH more than 5 is kept for at least 16–18 hours per day.

- In case of double resistance to metronidazole and clarithromycin, quadruple therapy is given by adding CBS to which resistance does not develop because it causes direct detachment of bacteria.

126. Why is domperidone preferred over metoclopramide? Explain.

- As domperidone does not cross BBB, it does not cause any extrapyramidal side effects which are very common with metoclopramide.
- It does not block therapeutic effect of levodopa and bromocriptine in idiopathic parkinsonism and counteracts their emetic action.
- Other side effects are much lesser than that of metoclopramide.
- Prokinetic action of domperidone is not attenuated by atropine.

127. Explain mechanism of action of domperidone/metoclopramide indicated in gastro-esophageal reflux disease (GERD).

- Majority of GERD patients present as functional defect, where in there is relaxation of lower esophageal sphincter in absence of swallowing.
- Repeated refluxes of acidic gastric contents into the lower 1/3rd of esophagus cause the manifestations like:
  - Heart burn
  - Sensation of food contents coming back into food pipe.

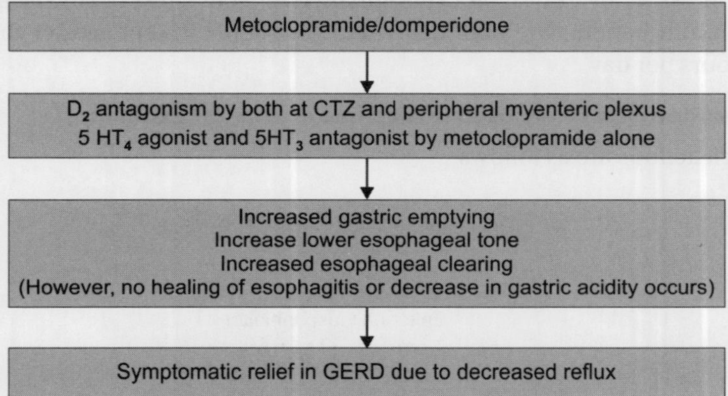

128. Why is ondansetron preferred in chemotherapy-induced vomiting? Explain.

- Ondansetron is a $5HD_3$ receptor antagonist, a prototype of a distinct glass of antiemetic drug to control cancer chemotherapy/radiotherapy-induced vomiting; caused due to damage at mucosal level (GI mucosa has a high-growth fraction).

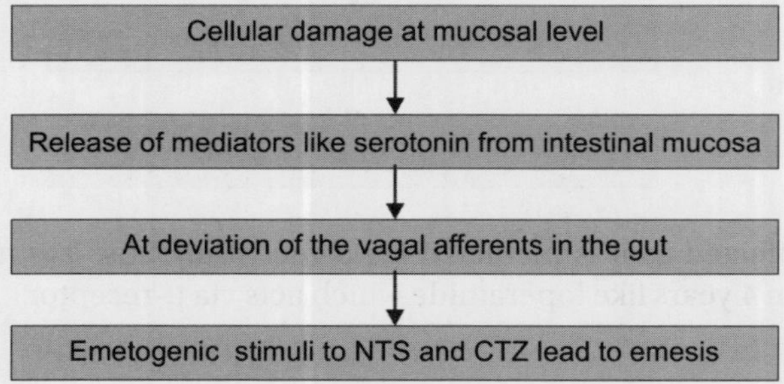

- Ondansetron blocks the depolarizing action of serotonin both through $5HT_3$ receptors on vagal afferents in the gut as well as in central nervous system (NTS and CTZ).
- This blocking emetogenic impulses both at their peripheral origin and their central relay prevents bio-amplification of the stimuli and proves most effective.
- Another mechanism of antiemesis is weak gastrokinetic action due to $5HT_3$ blockade, but is clinically insignificant.

129. What is the combination therapy used in *H. pylori* infection? Explain.

- Combination therapy used in *H. pylori* infection is triple therapy (omeprazole 40 mg OD + metronidazole 400 mg TDS + amoxicillin 500 mg TDS) or quadruple therapy (colloidal bismuth subcitrate (CBS) 20 mg QID + tetracycline 500 mg QID + metronidazole 400 mg TDS + omeprazole 20 mg BD).
- It is used as:
  - Eradication of *H. pylori* with H_2 blocker/PPI therapy of peptic ulcer has been associated with faster ulcer healing.
  - It largely prevents relapse and high rate of eradication.
  - To prevent development of resistance to single drug.
  - In quadruple therapy CBS is used not to develop drug resistance.
  - Acid suppression by PPI/H_2 blockers enhances effectiveness of anti-*H. pylori* antibiotics and optimum benefits are obtained when gastric pH is kept greater than 5 for at least 16–18 hours per day.

130. Can racecadotril be safely used in diarrhea in infants? Explain.

- Racecadotril actions are as follows:

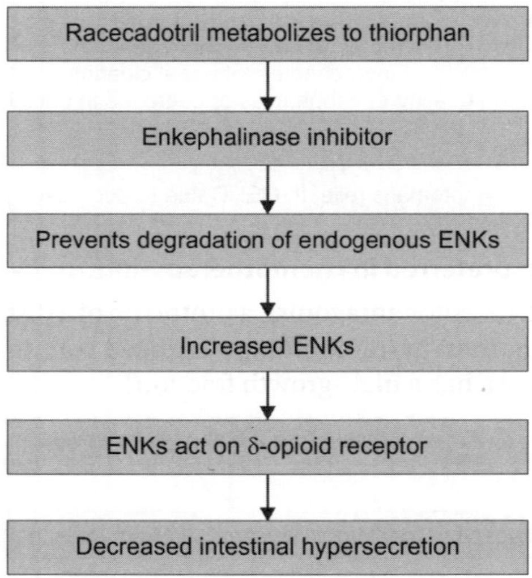

- Motility is not affected as it is mediated via μ-receptor. Thus, it is not contraindicated in children less than 4 years like loperamide which acts via μ-receptor.

131. Why are corticosteroids contraindicated in peptic ulcer? Explain.

- Corticosteroids inhibit prostaglandin synthesis. Thus, the ulcer protective effect of PG is gone.
- The ulcer protective effects of PG are:
  - Decreases acid secretion
  - Increases mucous secretion
  - Increases HCO_3^- secretion
  - Decreases gastrin secretion
  - Cytoprotective effect
  - Increases blood flow.
- Thus, corticosteroids are contraindicated in peptic ulcer.

ANTIMICROBIAL DRUGS

132. Explain mechanism of action of acyclovir as an antiviral agent.

- Acyclovir is a deoxy-guanosine analog antiviral drug that is mainly effective against HSV-1, HSV-2 and less effective in varicella zoster virus infection.

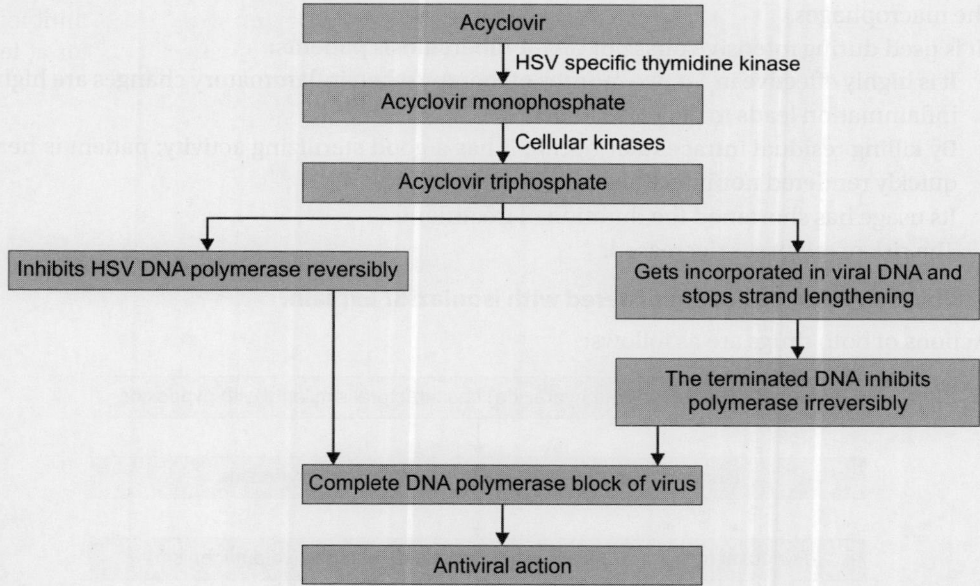

133. Why is primaquine used in *P. vivax* and *P. ovale* malaria? Explain.

- Unlike other antimalarial drugs, primaquine is a poor erythrocytic schizonticide and has weak action on *P. vivax* blood forms while *P. falciparum* blood forms are totally insensitive.
- It is more active against preerythrocytic stage of *P. falciparum* than *P. vivax*.
- The primary indication of primaquine is for radical cure of relapsing malaria (*P. vivax* and *P. ovale*), as it has strong activity against hypnozoites.

- So, along with a schizonticide, primaquine is given to reduce the possibility of relapse and also development of drug resistance.

134. Why should not penicillin and chloramphenicol be used together in meningitis patients? Explain.

- Penicillin is a bactericidal drug and chloramphenicol is bacteriostatic drug.
- If an organism is highly sensitive to the cidal action of a drug, response to the bactericidal—bacteriostatic combination is equal to the static drug given alone. This is known as "apparent antagonism". This happens because cidal drugs act primarily on rapidly multiplying bacteria, while static drugs retard multiplication.
- So, in the above case, pneumococci (causative agent of meningitis) is highly sensitive to penicillin and combination therapy of penicillin and chloramphenicol leads to higher patient mortality.

135. Why is pyrazinamide used during intensive phase of antitubercular therapy in CAT-1 patients? Explain.

- Pyrazinamide is weakly tuberculocidal and more active in acidic medium.
- It is more lethal to intracellularly located bacilli which lie within the acidic phagosome of the macrophages.
- It is used during intensive phase of CAT-1 tuberculosis patients:
  - It is highly effective in 1st two months of therapy when inflammatory changes are high as inflammation leads to decrease in pH.
  - By killing residual intracellular bacilli, it has a good sterilizing activity; patient is hence quickly rendered noninfectious.
  - Its usage has shortened the duration of treatment.
  - The risk of relapse is decreased.

136. Why is pyridoxine coadministered with isoniazid? Explain.

- Actions of both drugs are as follows:

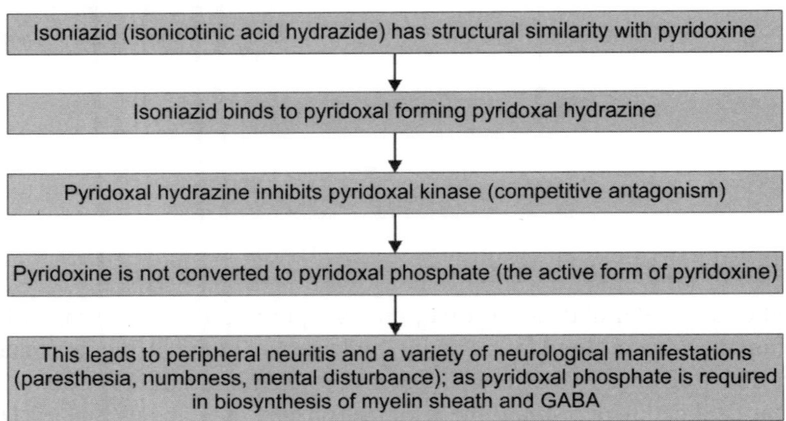

- So, pyridoxine is given prophylactically (10 mg/day) to prevent peripheral neuritis.

137. Why are aminoglycosides preferred in gram-negative aerobic infections? Explain.

- Transport of aminoglycoside into a bacterial cell is a multi-step process as follows:

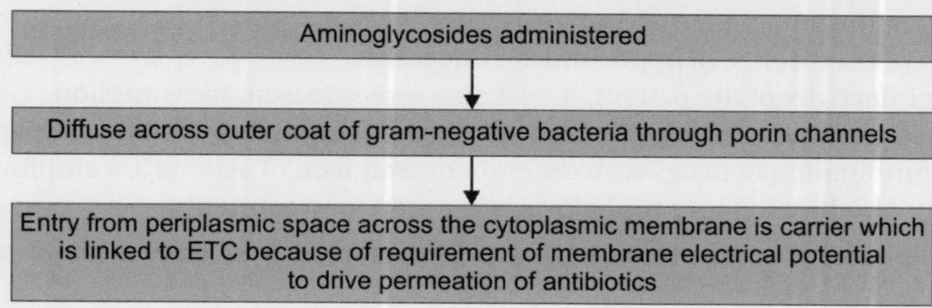

- Thus, penetration is dependent upon maintenance of a polarized membrane and on oxygen dependent active process. These are inactivated in anaerobic conditions and hence they are more effective in gram-negative aerobic bacteria.
- Moreover, augmentation of carrier mediated EDP-II entry present in gram-negative bacteria leads to more lethal action on microbes.

138. Why is rifampicin used once monthly in leprosy but frequent doses are required in pulmonary tuberculosis? Explain.

- Rifampicin capsule is given in leprosy once monthly, because:
  - *Mycobacterium leprae* is a very slowly multiplying organism; generation time is 12–14 days.
  - Single dose can kill 95–99% organisms.
  - Cost-benefit ratio is maximum.
- In *Mycobacterium tuberculosis,* rifampicin is used in frequent doses, because:
  - It is a very rapidly growing organism; generation time is 12–13 hours.
  - To kill rapidly subpopulations like rapid growing bacilli and spurters, frequent dosing is a must.

139. Why is a preparation of tazobactam + piperacillin is used in certain bacterial infections? Explain.

- This is because tazobactam is a beta-lactamase inhibitor and piperacillin is a ureidopenicillin.
- The antibacterial action of piperacillin is due to the presence of beta-lactam ring which is broken by beta-lactamase produced by some bacteria.
- Tazobactam by inhibiting beta-lactamase prevents destruction of piperacillin and potentiates its antimicrobial action. Thus, tazobactam acts as sentry drug in this combination.
- The pharmacokinetics of tazobactam and piperacillin are similar.
- Moreover, the block produced by tazobactam is initially reversible but later becomes covalent and irreversible, i.e. progressive block leading to suicide inhibition.

140. Why is a combination chemotherapy used in HAART regimen? Explain.

- In highly active antiretroviral therapy (HAART) regimen, drugs with different mechanism of action should be used.
- This leads to adding up of therapeutic beneficial effects without adding up of adverse effects.
- It usually contains a combination of 2 NRTI + 1NNRTI/ 1PI.

- The objectives are:
  - To suppress viral replication so the patient can attain and maintain effective immune response.
  - To prevent the emergence of drug resistance in virus.
  - To prevent occurrence of opportunistic infections.
  - To limit infectivity of the patient, thus it also serves to limit transmission.
- HIV virus is extremely mutagenic and no single drug therapy is effective against it. So, always a combination of drugs with different mechanism of actions are employed together.
- HAART can also be used for prophylaxis other than for treatment.

141. Why is liposomal amphotericin-B (Amp-B) preferred over conventional preparation? Explain.

- Liposomal Amp-B consists of 10% Amp-B incorporated in uniform (60-80 nm) unilamellar liposomes made up of lecithin and biodegradable phospholipids.
- They are preferred over conventional preparation because:
  - It has better tolerability in IV infusion, as it produces only mild acute reaction.
  - Site-specific drug delivery is achieved, i.e to the reticuloendothelial cells.
  - It can be used in patients not tolerating infusion of conventional Amp-B preparation.
  - It has lower anemia producing propensity.
  - It has lower nephrotoxicity.
  - Delivery of Amp-B to RE cells of liver and spleen is particularly effective for kala-azar and immune compromised patients.
- Dose that can be given without toxicity is much higher for liposomal Amp-B
  - *Conventional*: 0.7 mg/kg/day
  - *Liposomal*: 3–5 mg/kg/day.

142. Tolerance and bacterial resistance are not synonymous in pharmacology. Explain why?

- Tolerance refers to the requirement of a higher dose of a drug to produce a given response. It is a widely occurring adaptive biological phenomenon.
- On the other hand, resistance refers to unresponsiveness of a microorganism to an antimicrobial agent.
- Hence, it is obvious that the two terms are not synonymous.

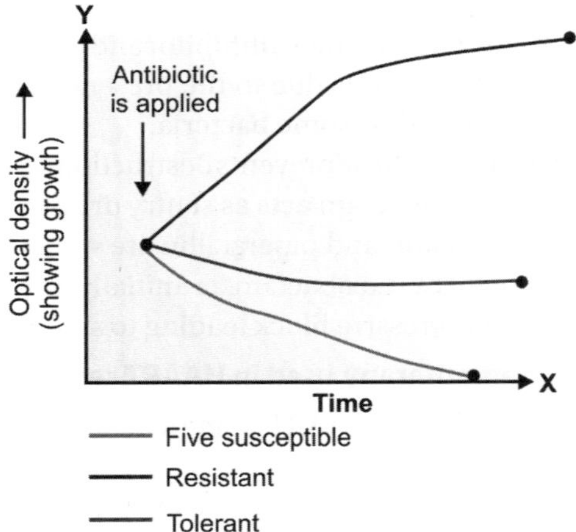

Fig. 6.10: Response to antibiotics: Susceptible vs Tolerant vs Resistant

143. Chloramphenicol should not be used in newborn babies. Explain why?

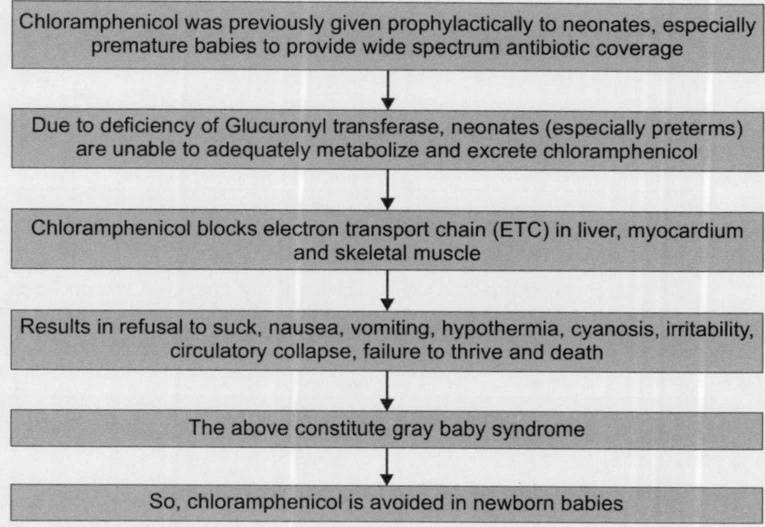

144. Urine should be alkalinized in sulfonamide therapy but acidified in methenamine therapy. Explain why?

- Sulfonamides are excreted partly unchanged and partly as acetylated byproduct. The acetylated product of sulfonamides are poorly soluble in acidic urine and may cause crystaluria, hematuria and even urinary tract obstruction. These can be avoided by alkalinizing urine in which both the excretory forms are more soluble.
- Methenamine is a pro drug (hexa-methylene-tetramine), which is degraded in acidic urine to release ammonia and formaldehyde which inhibit all bacteria. So, it is evident, that acidic urine is essential for its function. Urinary pH must be kept below 5.5 by administering organic acids like mandelic or hippuric acid concurrently with methenamine.

145. Why is multidrug therapy preferred in TB? Explain.

- WHO recommends the use of multidrug therapy for all cases of tuberculosis.
- The objectives are:
  - To make the patient noninfectious as early as possible by rapidly killing the dividing bacilli by using 3–4 bactericidal drugs.
  - To prevent the emergence of drug-resistant bacilli.
  - To prevent relapse by killing persisters (dormant population of *M.tuberculosis*).
  - To reduce total duration of effective therapy.
  - The dose of individual drugs is reduced, so there is less toxicity.
  - To equally kill all subpopulations of AFB like rapid growers, spurters, dormants, etc.
- The therapeutic effects are added up in the multidrug therapy but the adverse effects are not.

146. Explain mechanism of action of azoles used as an antifungals.

- Azoles are presently exclusively used as antifungal drugs.
- The mechanism of action of azole are as follows:

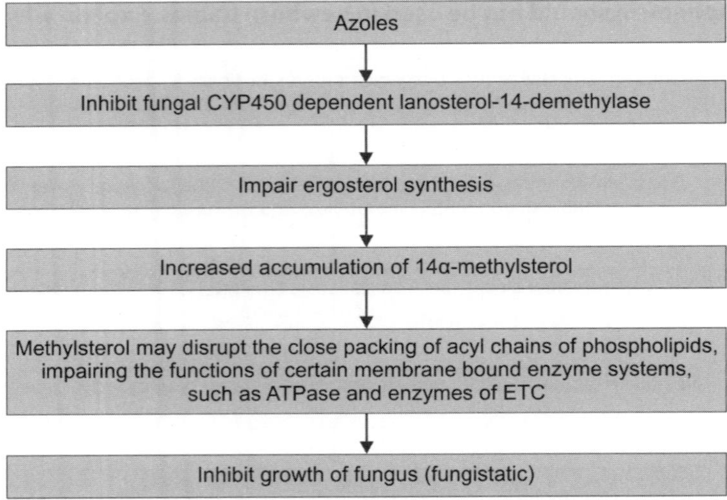

147. Explain mechanism of action of ACT in falciparum malaria.

- Artemisinin is a sesquiterpene-lactone-endoperoxide active against *Plasmodium falciparum* resistant to all other antimalarial drugs.
- It exerts potent and rapid blood schizonticide action.

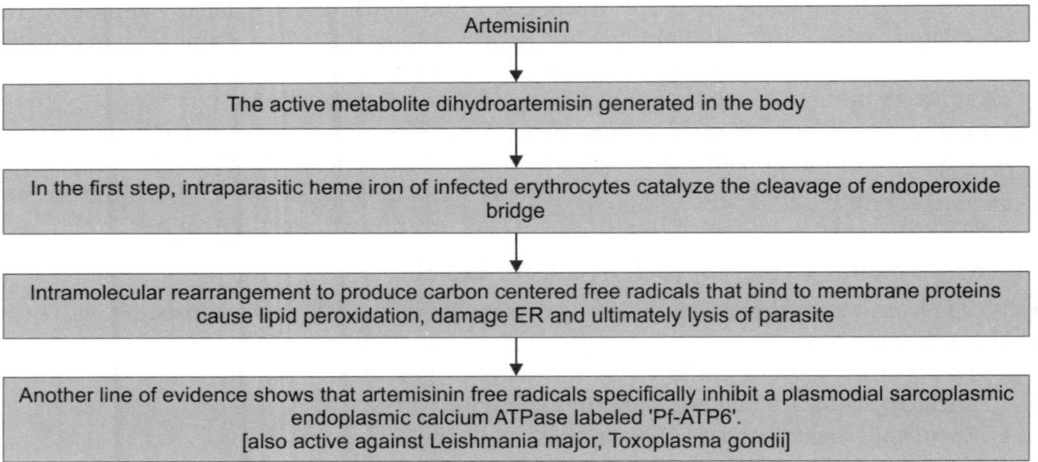

148. Explain mechanism of action of tetracyclines.

It is actively taken up by the susceptible bacteria, e.g. gram-negative bacteria tetracycline diffuse through porin channels and more lipid soluble members enter by passive diffusion

↓

Binds to reversibly 30s ribosomal subunit

↓

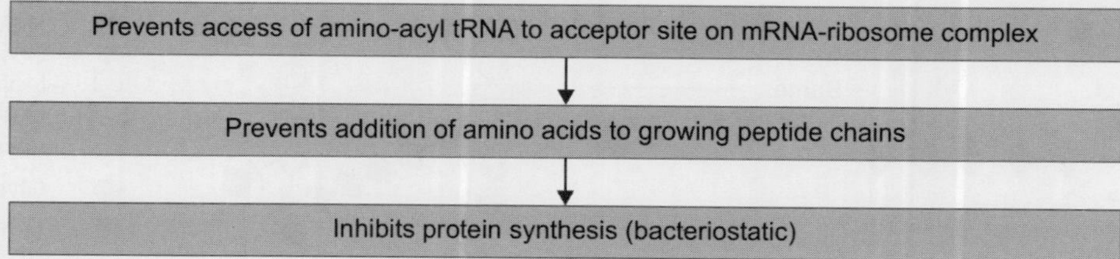

149. Explain mechanism of action of choroquine.

- It is rapidly acting erythrocytic schizonticide against all species of *Plasmodium.*
- Its mechanism of action of is as follows:

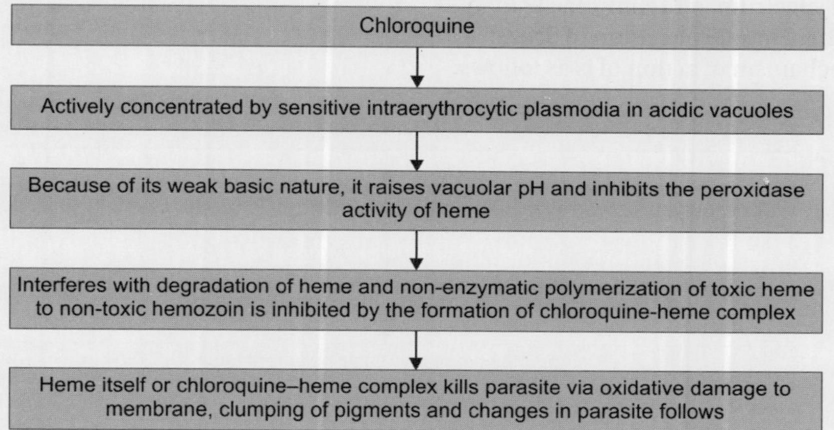

150. Explain mechanism of action of crystalline penicillin used as an antimicrobial.

- Crystalline penicillin/sodium-benzyl penicillin inhibits with the synthesis of bacterial cell wall.
- Its mechanism of action of is as follows:

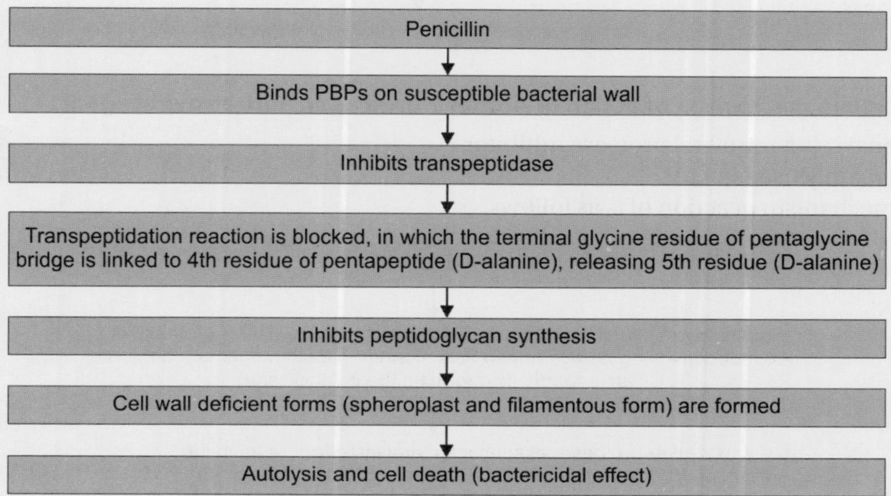

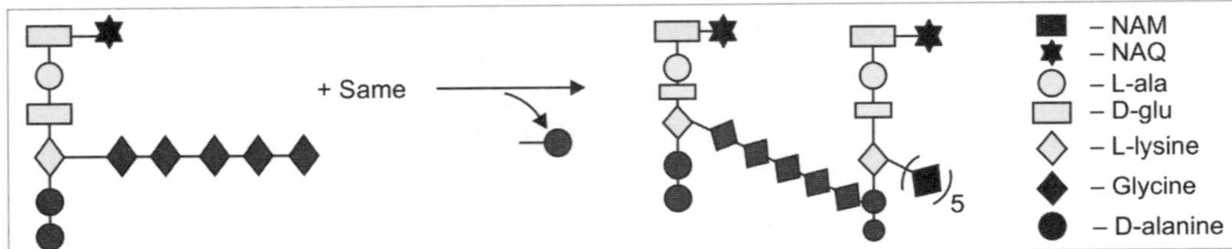

Fig. 6.11: MOA of penicillin at molecular level

151. Explain mechanism of action of albendazole as an antihelminthic.

- Broad spectrum anthelminthic activity.
- It is a benzimidazole group of drugs.
- Its mechanism of action of is as follows:

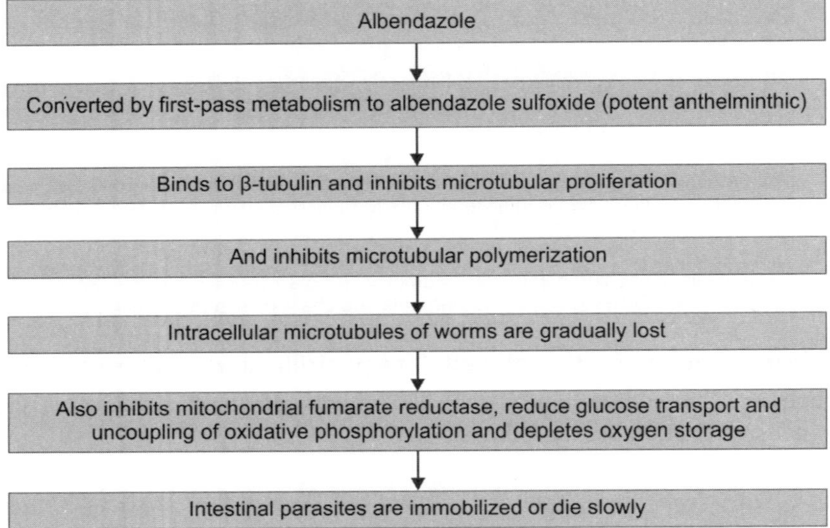

152. Explain mechanism of action of ritonavir used as an antiretroviral agent.

- Ritonavir is a retroviral protease inhibitor.
- It is mainly used in HIV.
- Its mechanism of action of is as follows:

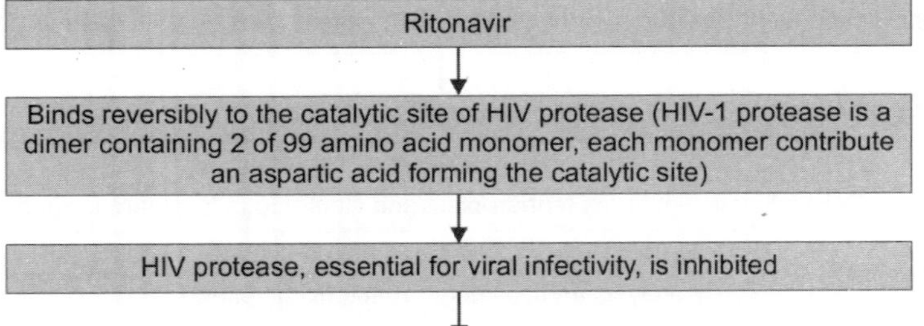

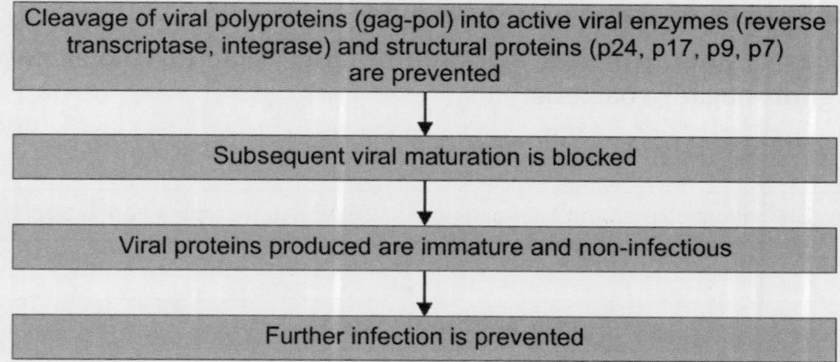

- Ritonavir boasted therapy, potent CYP3A4 inhibitor, improves compliance (6–18 tablets reduced to 2 tablets/day).
- In low and subthreshold dose (100 mg), increased bioavailability of companion PI by competing for presystemic metabolism and decreased clearance by competing for systemic metabolism.
- As they act at a late stage of viral maturation, they are effective in both newly and chronically effective cells.

153. Why is ciprofloxacin avoided in children? Explain.

- Ciprofloxacin is avoided in children as:
  - It is found that ciprofloxacin causes cartilage damage in weight bearing joints.
  - Arthralgia and joint swelling has been reported in many children receiving ciprofloxacin.

154. Explain mechanism of action of macrolide antibiotics.

- Macrolide antibiotics have a macrocyclic lactone ring with attached sugars.
- Its activity is enhanced in alkaline medium as non-ionized form of the drug is favored in higher pH.

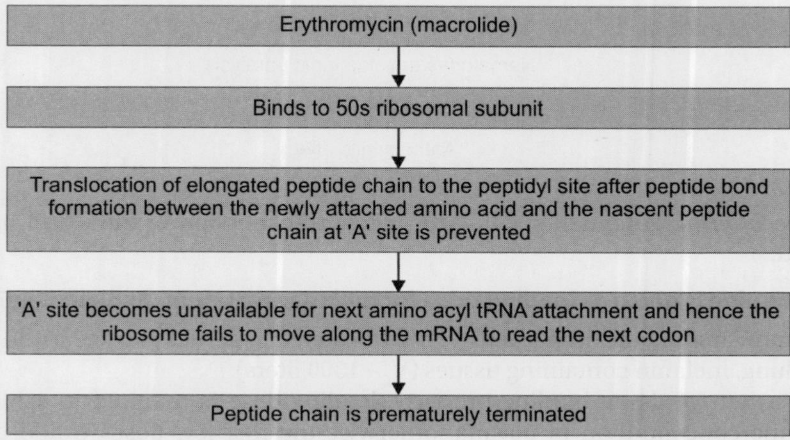

- It is seen that synthesis of larger proteins is selectively suppresses and this results in the antimicrobial activity.

155. Explain mechanism of action of sulfonamides

- They are a class of antimicrobials that are primarily bacteriostatic against many gram-positive and gram-negative bacteria.
- Its mechanism of action of is as follows:

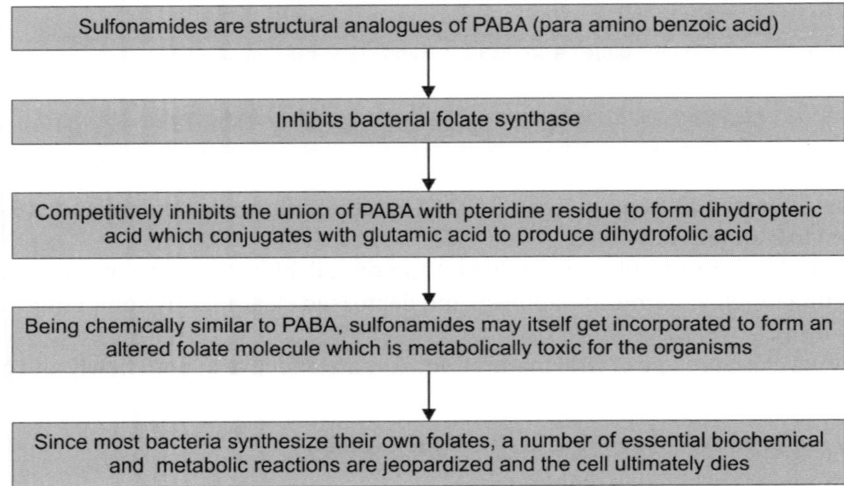

156. Explain mechanism of action of ivermectin as anthelminthic

- Ivermectin is an extremely potent semisynthetic derivative of the antinematodal principle obtained from *Streptomyces avermitilis*.
- Its mechanism of action of is as follows:

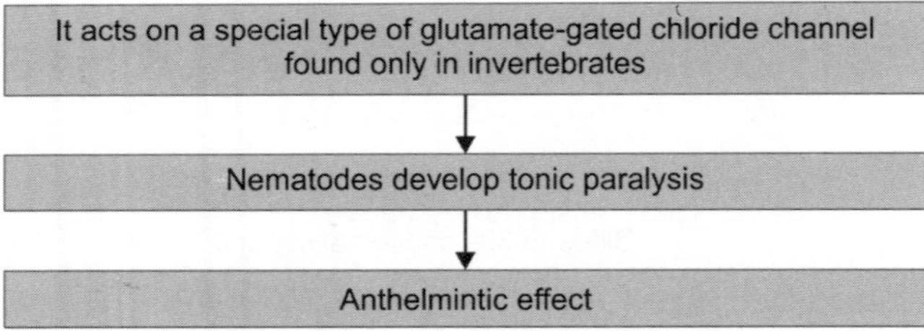

- *Other mechanism*: Potentiation of GABA-nergic transmission in the worm has also been observed.

157. Chloroquine is given as loading dose for malaria treatment. Explain why?

- After administration, the drug extensively sequestered in tissues particularly in liver, spleen, kidney, lung, melanin containing tissues (V_L ~ 1300 liters).
- For this extensive tissue-binding property, loading dose is required to achieve effective therapeutic concentration in plasma, otherwise the first few doses would be wasted in saturating the tissue binding sites.
  - Loading dose = (Target C_p X V)/F

- For chloroquine is 600 mg followed by 300 mg at 8 hours and then at 2nd and 3rd days OD.

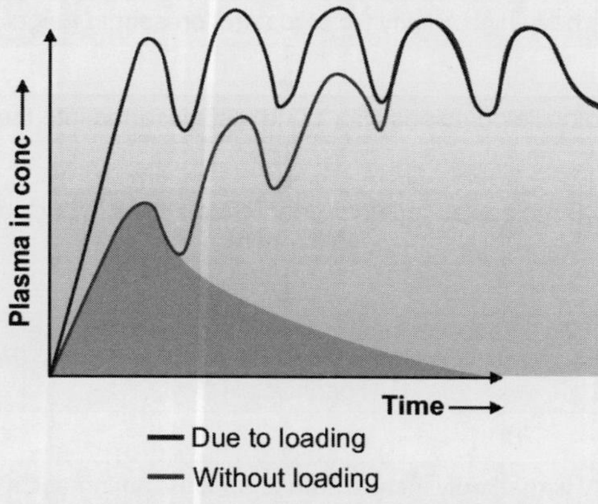

Fig. 6.12: Importance of loading dose of a drug

158. Aminoglycosides should not be used in pregnancy. Explain why?

- Aminoglycosides are potentially ototoxic (pregnancy drug category D).
- So, to avoid risk of fetal ototoxicity, aminoglycosides should not be used in pregnancy.

159. Doxycycline is the preferred over tetracycline. Explain why?

- It can be administered orally as well as intravenously.
- It is almost completely absorbed after oral administration (95–100%).
- Food does not interfere with its absorption.
- It has longer duration of action (half-life almost 24 hours).
- Diarrhea is rare, as it does not affect intestinal floras and very little amount reaches large gut in active form.
- It can be safely given to the patients with renal failure, as it is excreted primarily in bile.
- Highly lipid-soluble, so can passively diffuse into susceptible bacteria without carrier–increased potency.

160. Why is metronidazole combined with diloxanide furoate for intestinal amebiasis? Explain.

- Metronidazole is a prototype nitro-imidazole used for intestinal amebiasis. However, it is less effective in eradicating amebic cysts from the colon, as it is nearly completely absorbed from upper bowel.
- Diloxanide furoate is a highly effective luminal amebicide. It directly kills the trophozoites responsible for production of cysts and produces cure in asymptomatic cyst passers.

161. Explain mechanism of action of amphotericin B used as an antifungal.

- Amphotericin B is a polyene antifungal antibiotic obtained from *Streptomyces nodosus*. The polyene possesses a macrocyclic ring, one side of which has several conjugated double bonds and is highly lipophilic, while other side is hydrophilic with many–OH groups.

- Its mechanism of action of is as follows:

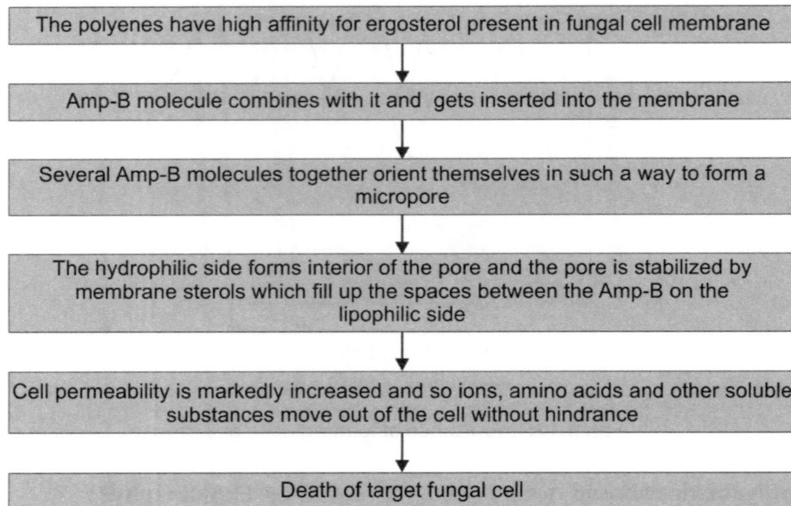

162. Explain mechanism of action of fluoroquinolones as an antimicrobial.

- These are synthetic antimicrobials having a quinolone structure that are active primarily against gram-negative bacteria, though the newer fluorinated compounds also inhibit gram-positive bacteria.
- Its mechanism of action of is as follows:

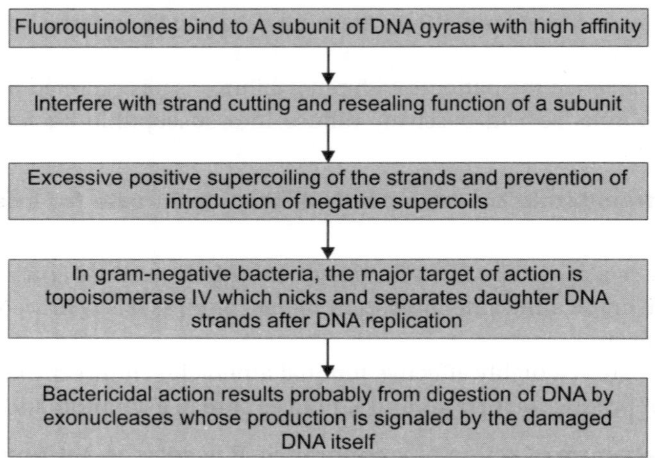

163. Why is fixed drug combination (FDC) used in cotrimoxazole? Explain.

- Cotrimoxazole is an FDC of trimethoprim and sulfamethoxazole.
- Mechanism of action is as follows:

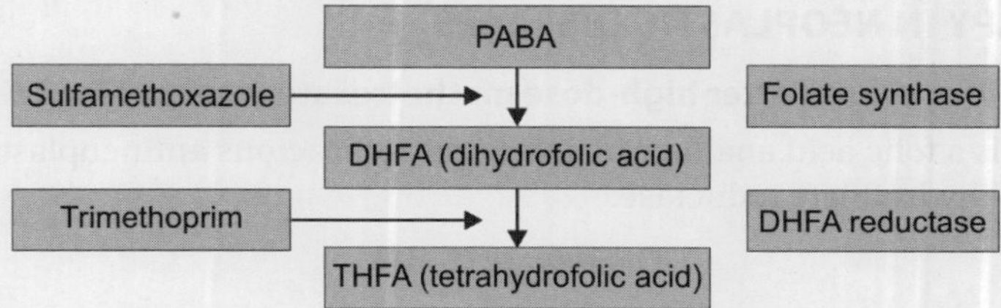

- The advantages of this combination are:
  - Sequential block produced by cotrimoxazole as shown above in folate synthesis is much more effective than individual drug block.
  - Both sulfamethoxazole and trimethoprim are bacteriostatic but the combination becomes cidal against many organisms.
  - Both drugs have similar half-life of about 10 hours.
  - Pharmacokinetics of drugs are such that when given in a dose ratio of 5:1, plasma concentration ratio of 20:1 is obtained (sulfamethoxazole: trimethoprim). This ratio produces maximum synergy such that MIC of each is reduced 3–6 times.

164. Explain mechanism of action of isoniazid (INH).

- The primary action of INH is inhibition of mycolic acid synthesis which makes it specific for *Mycobacterium tuberculosis.*
- Mechanism of action is as follows:

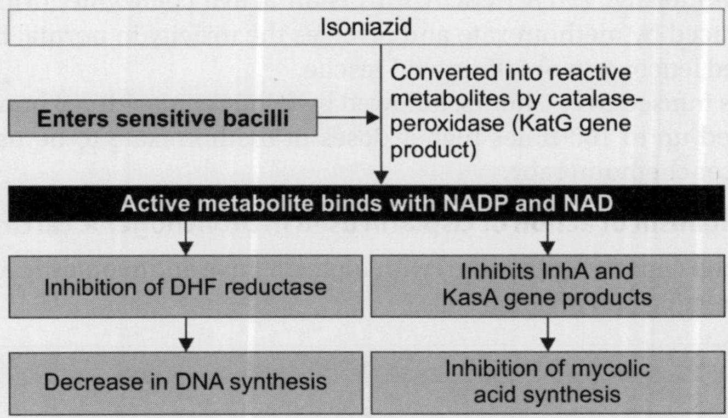

165. Why is probenecid used with penicillin? Explain.

- This is because probenecid blocks tubular secretion of penicillin by bidirectional block of OATP family of transporters in renal tubules. Thus, higher and long-lasting plasma concentration is achieved as penicillin is predominantly secreted and resorbed minimally from renal tubules.
- Probenecid also decreases the volume of distribution of penicillin which leads to higher steady-state plasma concentrations.

CHEMOTHERAPY IN NEOPLASTIC DISEASES

166. Why is folinic acid used after high-dose methotrexate therapy? Explain.

- Methotrexate is a folic acid analog which is highly efficacious antineoplastic drug and acts by inhibiting dihydrofolate reductase:

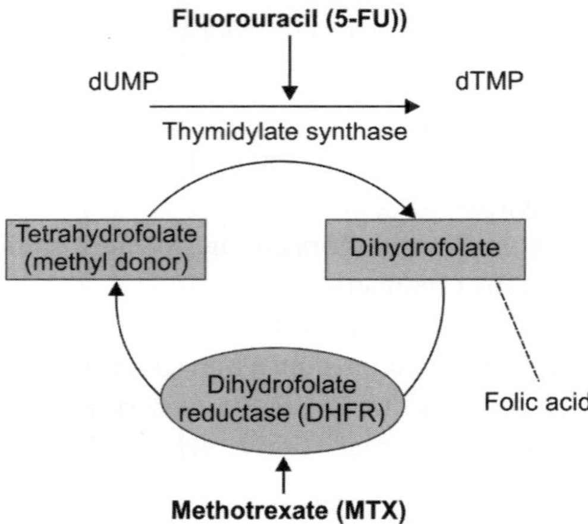

Fig. 6.13: Mechanism of action of Mtx & 5FU

- To reduce the toxicity of methotrexate like bone marrow suppression, immune suppression and megaloblastic anemia, folinic acid is administered.
- Folinic acid (N-5 formyl THFA /leucovorin) is an active coenzyme form which bypasses the block produced by methotrexate and reverses the toxicity in normal body tissues. This method is called leucovorin or folinic acid rescue.
- Methotrexate is infused over 6 hours, followed by folinic acid within 3 hours.
- This has allowed up to 100 times higher doses of methotrexate to be used for increased efficacy of cancer chemotherapy.

167. Explain mechanism of action of cisplatin used in bronchogenic carcinoma.

- It is a heavy metal complex (platinum) with high effective antineoplastic activity.
- It acts both on resting and dividing cells.

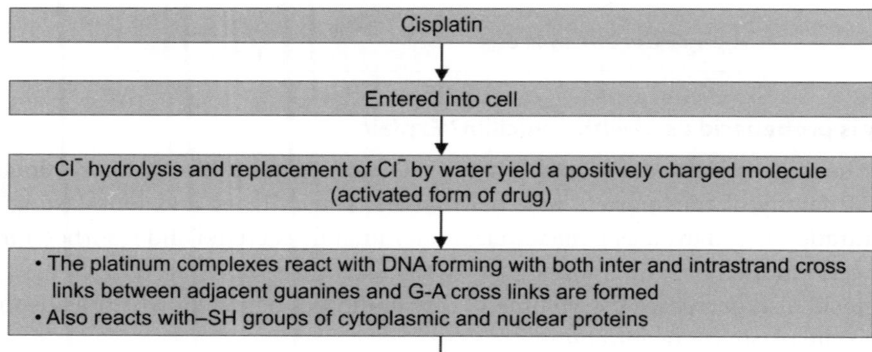

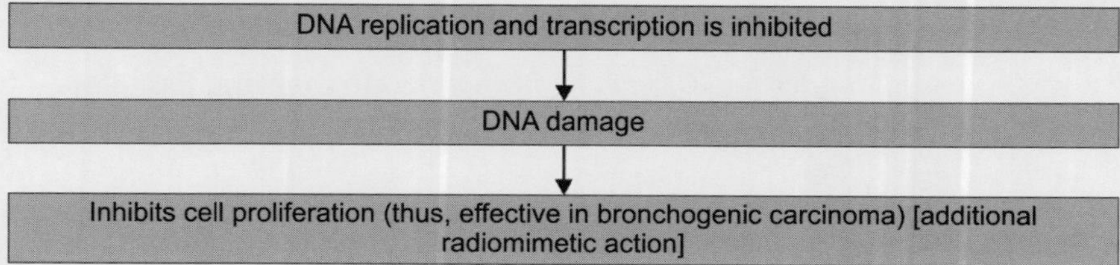

168. Why is antineoplastic therapy given in cancer cell cycles? Explain.

- The use of antineoplastic therapy in pulses allows the noncycling population of cancer cells to reenter the cell cycle in-between drug courses, thus allowing better and complete cure.
- The most important target of action of cytotoxic anticancer drugs are nucleic acid and their precursors and rapid nucleic acid synthesis during cell division.

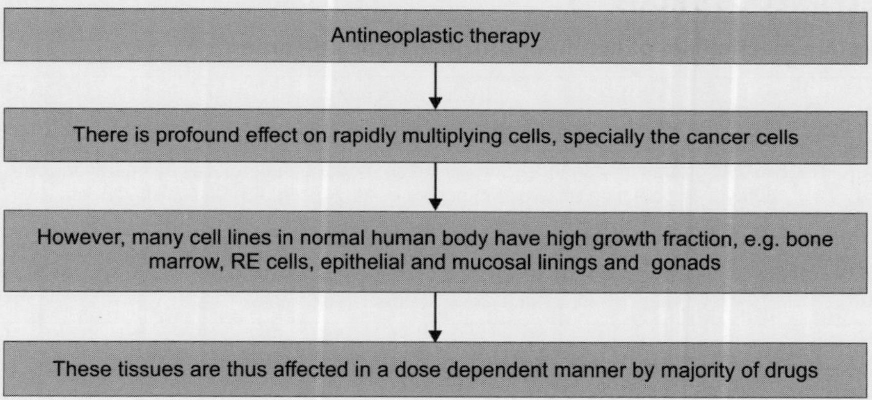

- The cyclic administration of these drugs allow the normal tissues to recover from cytotoxic assault.
  - Cycling allows "kinetic scheduling" of the drugs: Cell cycle specific drugs are generally scheduled after a course of cell cycle nonspecific drugs to improve cell kill.
  - Cycling of drugs does not allow resistance to develop easily.
  - Interval between chemotherapy cycles may be used for other treatment forms like radiation therapy.
  - Better patient compliance then continuous therapy.
  - Fraction kill hypothesis:
    - Considering a tumor of 10^{11} cells and 99% kill per cycle of chemotherapy; cell no would be reduced to <1 in 6 chemo cycles because ($0.01^{6} = 10^{-12}$)
    - Some regrowth occurs during the rest interval but the rate of cell kill exceeds the rate of regrowth.

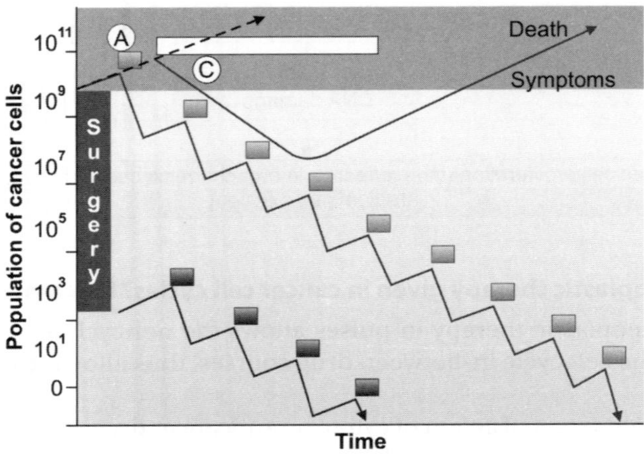

Fig. 6.14: Fraction kill hypothesis of cancer therapy

MISCELLANEOUS DRUGS

169. Explain mechanism of action of BAL in arsenic poisoning.

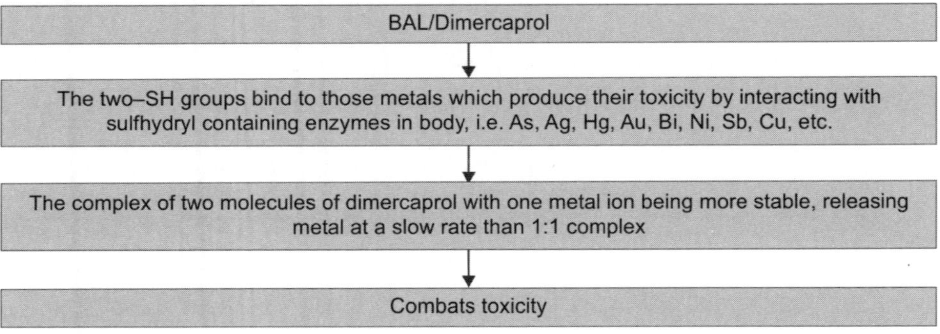

170. Why is penicillamine used in Wilson's disease? Explain.

- Penicillamine is chemically dimethyl cysteine, obtained as a degradation product of penicillin.
- Its actions are as follows:

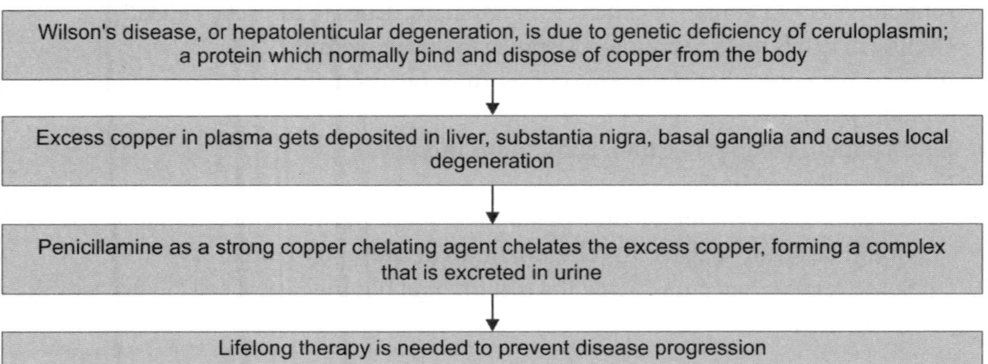

171. Why is desferrioxamine used in thalassemia? Explain.

- Desferrioxamine is an iron chelating agent which has very high affinity for iron, i.e. 1g is capable of chelating 85 mg of elemental iron.
- It removes loosely bound iron as well as from hemosiderin and ferritin but nor from hemoglobin or cytochrome.

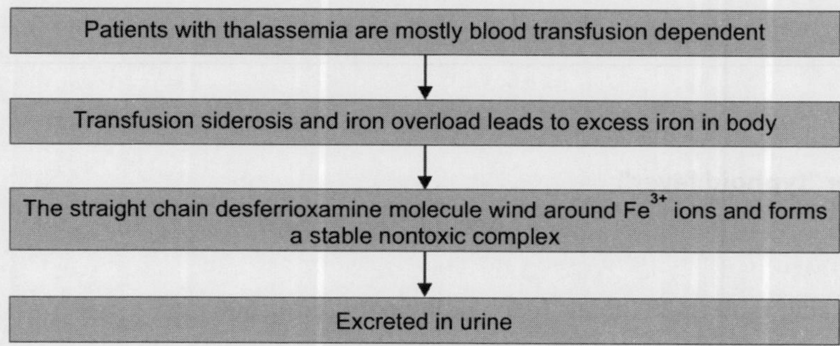

- Desferrioxamine 0.5–1 mg per day IM helps excrete chronic iron overload. It may also be infused concurrently with blood transfusion (2 g/unit of whole blood).

CHAPTER 7

Prescription Writing

Arnab Pal

1. A drug for "typhoid fever".

For Mr X Age: Sex:

R_x

Ciprofloxacin tablets: 28 tablets (each tablet containing 500 mg)

Direction: One tablet to be taken twice daily after meal for 2 weeks.

Date: ________________ ABC

VIVA

1. Others drugs used in typhoid fever?

2. A drug for "bacillary dysentery".

For Mr X Age: Sex:

R_x

Norfloxacin tablets: 10 tablets (each tablet containing 400 mg)

Direction: One tablet to be taken twice daily after meal for 5 days.

Date: ________________ ABC

VIVA

1. Dysentery vs diarrhea.
2. Other drugs used.

3. A drug for "duodenal ulcer".

For Mr X, Age: Sex:

R_x

Ranitidine tablets: 42 tablets (each tablet containing 300 mg)

Direction: One tablet to be taken once daily at bedtime for 6 weeks.

Date: ________________ ABC

VIVA

1. Proton pump inhibitors (PPI) vs H_2 blockers.
2. Other drugs used.

3. Advantage of H_2 blockers of PPI.
4. Advantage of PPI over H_2 blockers.

4. A drug for "amebic dysentery".

For Mr X Age Sex:

R_x

Metronidazole tablets: 21 tablets (each tablet containing 400 mg)

Direction: One tablet to be thrice twice daily for 7 days.

Date: ________________ ABC

VIVA

1. Where is 800 mg TDS dose used?

5. A drug for "tonic-clonic seizures".

For Mr X Age: Sex:

R_x

Phenytoin sodium tablets: 24 tablets (each tablet containing 100 mg)

Direction: One tablet to be taken thrice daily and the patient must report after 7 days.

Date: ________________ ABC

VIVA

1. Drugs used to treat epilepsy.
2. Define epilepsy.
3. Side effects and pharmacokinetics of phenytoin.
4. What is catamenial epilepsy?

6. A drug for "multibacillary leprosy".

For Mr X Age: Sex:

R_x

1. Rifampicin capsules
   (Each capsule containing 600 mg)
   Direction: One capsule to be taken 1 hour before breakfast once a month (supervised).
2. Dapsone tablets
   (Each tablet containing 100 mg)
   Direction: One tablet to be taken daily after breakfast.
3. Clofazimine capsules
   (Each capsule containing 50 mg)
   Direction: One capsule to be taken daily and six capsules to be taken once a month (supervised).

The above regimen is to be continued for 1 year duration.

Date: ________________ ABC

VIVA

1. Why monthly rifampicin in leprosy but daily in tuberculosis (TB)?

7. A drug for "Taeniasis".

For Mr X Age: Sex:

R_x

Miconazole ointment (2%): 1 tube (each tube containing 15 gm)

Direction: The ointment is to be applied over affected areas twice daily for 1 month.

Date: ________________ ABC

VIVA

1. Types of taeniasis.
2. Enumerate topical antifungal drugs.
3. Drugs used against dermatophytes.

8. A drug for "urinary tract infection".

For Mr X Age: Sex:

R_x

Norfloxacin tablets: 28 tablets (each tablet containing 400 mg)

Direction: One tablet to be taken twice daily after meal for 2 weeks.

Date: ________________ ABC

VIVA

1. Other drugs for urinary tract infection (UTI).
2. Use of phenazopyridine in UTI.

9. A drug for "acute bacterial conjunctivitis".

For Mr X Age: Sex:

R_x

Ciprofloxacin eye drop: 1 vial (each vial containing 5 mL, 0.3% of the drug)
Ciprofloxacin eye ointment: 1 tube (each tube containing 5 g, 0.3% of the drug)

Direction: Two drops of the eyedrop to be instilled in each eye three times daily during the day time and the ointment should be applied to the inner aspect of lower eyelid at bed time till condition improves.

Date: ________________ ABC

10. A drug for "filariasis".

For Mr X Age: Sex:

R_x

Diethylcarbamazine citrate tablets: 63 tablets (Each tablet containing 100 mg)

Direction: One tablet to be taken thrice daily for 21 days.

Date: ________________ ABC

VIVA

1. Other drugs used.

11. A drug for "acute gout".

For Mr X Age: Sex:

R_x

Colchicine tablets: 06 tablets (each tablet containing 0.5 mg)

Direction: Two tablets to be taken immediately followed by one tablet every 2 hourly until relief of pain is obtained or vomiting or diarrhea results.

Date: ________ ABC

VIVA

1. What are disease-modifying antirheumatic drugs (DMARDs)?
2. What is the vicious cycle of gout?

12. A drug for "nausea and vomiting".

For Mr X Age: Sex:

R_x

Metoclopramide tablets: 02 tablets (each tablet containing 10 mg)

Direction: One tablet to be taken immediately and the other to be repeated if necessary.

Date: ________ ABC

VIVA

1. Side effects of metoclopramide.
2. Other uses of this drug.
3. Other antiemetics.

13. A drug for "mixed worm infestation".

For Mr X Age: Sex:

R_x

Mebendazole tablets: 06 tablets (Each tablet containing 100 mg)

Direction: One tablet to be taken twice daily for three consecutive days.

Date: ________ ABC

Or

For Mr X Age: Sex:

R_x

Albendazole tablet: 01 tablet (each tablet containing 400 mg)

Direction: One tablet to be taken after dinner preferably after fatty meal.

Date: ________ ABC

VIVA

1. Drugs used in neurocysticercosis.

14. A drug for "migraine".

For Mr X Age: Sex:

R_x

Sumatriptan tablets: 02 tablets (each tablet containing 50 mg)

Direction: One tablet to be taken immediately during the attack and the other to be repeated if necessary after 2 hours.

Date: ________________ ABC

Or

For Mr X Age: Sex:

R_x

(Ergometrine + Caffeine) tablets: 06 tablets (Each tablet containing ergometrine 1 mg and caffeine 100 mg)

Direction: One tablet to be taken immediately and followed by one tablet every half hourly if necessary; till relief of pain is obtained.

Date: ________________ ABC

VIVA

1. Drugs used in migraine prophylaxis.
2. Pathophysiology of migraine.

15. A drug for "syphilis".

For Mr X Age: Sex:

R_x

1. Benzathine penicillin: 1 vial containing 2.4 million units
2. Water for injection: 1 ampoule (each ampoule containing 5 mL)

Direction: Contents of the vial to be dissolved in 3 mL of water for injection and half of the amount is to be injected with a wide bore needle deep intramuscularly in each buttock.

Date: ________________ ABC

16. A drug for "gonorrhea".

For Mr X Age: Sex:

R_x

1. Amoxicillin capsules: 6 capsules (each capsule containing 500 mg)
   Direction: All the six capsules to be taken at a time.
2. Probenecid tablets: 2 tablets (each tablet containing 500 mg)
   Direction: Two tablets to be taken half an hour before administration of capsules.

Date: ________________ ABC

17. A drug for "acute attack of angina pectoris".

For Mr X Age: Sex:

R_x

Glyceryl trinitrate tablets: 03 tablets (each tablet containing 0.5 mg)

Direction: One tablet to be taken sublingually during the attack and the other when necessary.

Date: ________________ ABC

VIVA

1. Other antianginals including newer drugs.
2. Types of angina and their pathophysiology.

18. A drug for "uncomplicated pulmonary tuberculosis".

For Mr X Age: Sex:

R_x

1. Isoniazid tablets: 180 tablets (each tablet containing 300 mg)
   Direction: one tablet to be taken daily before breakfast for 6 months.
2. Rifampicin capsules: 180 capsules (each capsule containing 450 mg)
   Direction: one tablet to be taken daily one hour before breakfast for 6 months.
3. Ethambutol tablets: 60 tablets (each tablet containing 800 mg)
   Direction: One tablet to be taken daily after breakfast for initial 2 months.
4. Pyrazinamide tablets: 120 tablets (each tablet containing 750 mg)
   Direction: Two tablets to be taken daily after breakfast for initial 2 months.
5. Pyridoxine hydrochloride tablets: 180 tablets (each tablet containing 10 mg)
   Direction: One tablet to be taken daily with isoniazid for 6 months.

Date: ________________ ABC

VIVA

1. First- and second-line drugs.
2. Multidrug-resistant (MDR) and extensively drug-resistant tuberculosis (XDR-TB).
3. Indications of corticosteroid in TB.
4. Changes in regimen for coexistent human immunodeficiency virus (HIV).

19. Prescribe a purgative.

For Mr X Age: Sex:

R_x

Bisacodyl tablets: 2 tablets (each tablet containing 5 mg)

Direction: Two tablets to be taken together at bedtime.

Date: ________________ ABC

VIVA

1. Purgative vs laxative.

CHAPTER 8

Prescription Criticism

Avishek Layek

DEFINITION

A prescription is a written order from a registered medical practitioner containing one or more medicines together with the directions of preparation and dispensation to the pharmacist and mode of administration for the patient (Table 8.1).

PARTS OF A COMPLETE PRESCRIPTION

1. *Patient's particulars*: Name, age, and sex.
2. *Superscription*: R_x or Recipe, meaning "take thou" or "you take." Another lesser accepted theory is that it is actually a prayer for well-being to God Jupiter.
3. *Inscription*: This the body of the prescription which consists of the generic names and amounts of the following:
   - Chief ingredient
   - Adjuvant or secondary drug (if any)
   - Corrigents or correctives (if any): To correct undesirable quality or action of chief ingredient (e.g. antiemetics to counteract emesis expected during antineoplastic chemotherapy).
   - Vehicle or excipient: To give suitable form of administration (e.g. spacer for bronchodilators in a patient with inappropriate hand-mouth coordination).
4. *Subscription*: Direction to the dispenser.
5. *Signature or transcription*: Direction to the patient.
6. *Initial of the prescriber*: Usually accompanied by registration number of the prescriber.
7. *Date* (of great medicolegal importance).

Table 8.1: Types of prescription

S. No.	*Precompounded prescription*	*Extemporaneous prescription*
1.	Contains drugs that are available in precompounded dosage forms, e.g. paracetamol 500 mg tablet	Contains ingredients of the drug in specified quantity along with directions of preparation, e.g. mixing 09% normal saline (1 part) with 10% dextrose (4 parts) for parenteral nutrition of neonates
2.	Pharmacists/nursing staff dispense the drugs wholly as manufactured	Ingredients of the drug are mixed in advised proportions and then dispensed as directed
3.	Used more often in recent times	Use restricted to intensive care units and certain dermatological preparations
4.	Safer and more quality assured	Associated with higher risk of contamination

Example of a Model Prescription

For Mr X, 20 years, Male *Patient's particulars*

R_x

Quinine Sulfate	0.3 g	Basis	}
Sulfuric acid	0.6 mL	Adjuvant	}
Syrup of Orange	4.0 mL	Corrigent	}
Chloroform Water	30 mL	Vehicle	} *Inscription*

Mix and make a dose mixture, send 6 such *Subscription*

One dose thrice daily

Signature or Transcription

Date: XYZ

(Initials)

Commonly Used Abbreviations in Prescriptions

AC	=	Before food
PC	=	After food
BD/BID	=	Twice daily
QD/QID/QDS	=	Four times daily
TD/TDS	=	Thrice daily
OD	=	Daily
SOS	=	When necessary
STAT	=	Immediately

POINTS TO NOTE FOR CRITICISM OF A PRESCRIPTION

1. Errors in format of the prescription (compare format with model prescription earlier).
   Examples:
   - Date missing
   - Improper directions to pharmacist or patient
   - Patient's particulars missing
   - Never to use numbers for dosing; always use words (e.g. two tablets instead of 2 tablets) as it prevents tampering.
2 Errors in drugs prescribed.
   Examples:
   - Any contraindications missed like sodium-glucose cotransporter 2 (SGLT2) inhibitors in type 1 or gestational diabetes mellitus (GDM).
   - Drugs having harmful interactions prescribed together like insulin and beta blocker.
   - Drugs having antagonism prescribed together like bacteriostatic and bactericidal antimicrobial agent (AMA) together.
   - The prescribed drug is not the drug of choice like domperidone used in motion sickness in place of scopolamine.
   - Wrong dose prescribed, like low dose aspirin as anti-inflammatory or not adjusting the dose of a drug as required in hepatic/renal compromise.
   - Wrong timing, like proton pump inhibitor after food, etc.

AN EXAMPLE OF PRESCRIPTION CRITICISM

1. *The prescription made for a school going child of known beta thalassemia.*

For Subham, Male

R_x

Tablet iron and folic acid (100 mg elemental iron and 500 µg folic acid)
One tablet to be taken thrice daily

ABCD

Criticism

Format Errors

Age of patient missing, date missing, and the registration number of the doctor is missing.

Drug-related Errors

Anemia or thalassemia is to be treated by regular blood transfusion along with iron chelators. Supplemental iron folic acid therapy is contraindicated.

Solution

To advise regular blood transfusion according to hemoglobin (Hb) levels with proper iron chelation therapy [intravenous (IV) or oral].

2. *The prescription of a known diabetic woman who has recently had urine pregnancy test positive.*

For Mrs Srishti, 28 Female

R_x

Tablet Linagliptin 5 mg
One tablet to be taken once daily after dinner.

Date: 03.07.2017.

Criticism

Format Errors

Initials and registration number of prescriber are missing.

Drug-related Errors

Sodium-glucose cotransporter 2 inhibitors (e.g. linagliptin) are contraindicated in pregnancy.

Solution

For all practical purposes, diabetes of pregnancy is to be treated with appropriate insulin regimen (split mixed or basal-bolus regimen). Other than that, metformin is the only oral antidiabetic agent which is safe for use in pregnancy both singly or in combination with insulin.

CHAPTER

9

Therapeutic Problems

Arnab Pal

1. A 10-year-old school girl suffering from mild exercise induced bronchial asthma have been treated with a metered dose inhaler containing 500 µg of Terbutaline per inhalation as and when required, which effectively controls the individual attack. However, she has attacks of wheezing every 3–4 weeks occurring during exercise even after above treatment schedule.

What treatment should now be given to reduce the frequency of attacks?

EXERCISE INDUCED BRONCHIAL ASTHMA

Presenting Features

Attacks of wheezing every 3–4 weeks occurring during exercise, even after treatment with Terbutaline.

Relevant Information

A 10-year-old school girl suffering from mild exercise induced bronchial asthma was effectively controlled by 500 mg Terbutaline inhalation as and when required.

Inference

As the girl even after treatment with Terbutaline inhalation has been experiencing attacks of wheezing during exercise; the said treatment schedule is not adequate and she needs additional drugs to added to her regime.

Treatment

- To continue Terbutaline 500 µg by inhalation as and when required
- Cromolyn sodium 5–10 mg 4 times daily by inhalation for 6–8 weeks and the patient is advised to report after 6–8 weeks.
- After 6–8 weeks, if the frequency of attacks remain unaltered then beclomethasone dipropionate 100 µg 4 times has to advise via inhalation used.

2. A 16-year-old girl has admitted to the emergency department with severe short of breath. She is diagnosed as acute bronchial asthma. She has been using metered dose inhalation of Salbutamol, Ipratropium and beclomethasone. In spite of the above treatment, the present attack is not controlled. What will be her immediate treatment?

ACUTE EXACERBATIONS OF BRONCHIAL ASTHMA

Presenting Features

Patient is having severe shortness of breath and she is admitted to emergency department.

Relevant Information

A 16-year-old girl has been using metered dose inhalation of Salbutamol, Ipratropium and Beclomethasone.

Inference

In spite of the treatment by above 3 drugs, she has developed an acute exacerbation of bronchial asthma.

Treatment

- Moist oxygen inhalation (2–3L/min) given before, during and after administration of bronchodilators to avoid worsening of ventilation-Perfusion mismatch.
- Inhalation of Salbutamol 5 mg or Terbutaline 10 mg by nebulizer or metered dose inhaler with spacer.
- Alternatively, Salbutamol 250 µg by slow i.v injection or Terbutaline 250–500 µg by s.c route.
- Aminophylline 5 mg/kg by slow i.v injection over 20 min may be administered to speed up the response.
- Hydrocortisone sodium succinate 200–500 mg i.v 6 hourly
- I.V. fluids slow infusion with 5% Dextrose-Saline
- Potassium supplement to correct hypokalemia produced by repeated doses of Salbutamol/ Terbutaline
- Alkalinization by i.v. Sodium bicarbonate to correct acidosis and to increase sensitivity to Bronchodilators
- *Antibiotics*: Amoxicillin (500 mg)+ Clavunilic acid 8 hourly.

3. A 69 years old woman suffering from congestive heart failure has been treated with 0.25 mg Digoxin tablet daily for last 3 months. But the heart failure is not controlled adequately.

What will be the treatment to control the heart failure adequately?

CONGESTIVE HEART FAILURE

Presenting Features

Inadequate control of congestive cardiac failure.

Relevant Information

A 69-year-old woman suffering from CCF has been treated with 0.25 mg digoxin tablet daily for last 3 months.

Inference

As the CCF is not adequately controlled by 0.25 mg digoxin daily alone; she needs additional treatment.

Treatment

A. *General measures*
- Physical rest
- Moderate salt restriction (2-3 gm/day) – no added salt
- Weight loss in obese patients
- Fluid and free water restriction (<1.5L/day); specially if hyponatremic

B. *Specific measures*
- Digoxin 0.25 mg tablet daily to be continued
- Frusemide 20–80 mg/day tablet to be added
- Enalapril tablet. Therapy to be started with low dose: 2.5 mg/daily and is to be given after stopping diuretic for 1–2 days. If there is no hypotension, the dose is gradually increased to maximum 40 mg/day after 3–4 days depending on the response
- Cause of heart failure is to be investigated and treated if possible.
- Serum K^+ is to be estimated at regular intervals and supplementation to be done accordingly.

4. A 45-year-old male patient with history of smoking presented with exertional retrosternal compressing pain radiating to the left arm and lasts for 2–5 minutes. The pain is relieved after taking rest. After proper investigation, he has been diagnosed as a case of stable angina pectoris. What will be the treatment to control the attack?

STABLE ANGINA

Presenting Features

Exertional retrosternal compressing pain radiating to the left arm, lasting for 2–5 mins and relieved by rest.

Relevant Information

A 45-year-old male patient with history of smoking.

Inference

The patient is diagnosed to be a case of stable angina pectoris and he needs treatment for control of acute attack and also for prevention for attacks.

Treatment

- The patient is advised to stop smoking
- Fat restricted diet
- For termination of acute attack: Glyceryl trinitrate Tablet 0.5 mg sublingually; maximum 3 tablets can be taken at 5 minutes interval.
- For prophylaxis:
  - Isosorbide mononitrate: 20 mg tablet, 1 tablet twice daily
  - Atenolol 50–100 mg tablet: once daily
  - Nifedipine 5–10 mg tablet, thrice daily initially and then gradually increased to 10-20 mg thrice daily.
  - Aspirin 75–150 mg tablet, once daily.

5. A 45-old-patient suffering from angina pectoris was on treatment with isosorbide dinitrate. He is admitted to the hospital with severe chest pain and sweating and diagnosed to be a case of acute myocardial infarction. What will be the management of this patient?

ACUTE MYOCARDIAL INFARCTION

Relevant Information

A 45-old-patient suffering from angina pectoris was on treatment with isosorbide dinitrate. He is admitted to the hospital with severe chest pain and sweating.

Inference

The patient is diagnosed to be a case of acute myocardial infarction.

Treatment

- General Measures
  - Patient is admitted to ICCU. Continuous monitoring of ECG, pulse oximetry and blood pressure to be done. Patient to be kept for at least 12 hours of complete bed rest
  - Supplemental moist oxygen therapy (4-6 L/min) is given if $SpO_2 < 90\%$. Mechanical ventilation if necessary
  - Ensure i.v access for drug administration
- Specific Treatment
  - Tablet Aspirin- 150–325 mg orally administered (to be chewed) and continued once daily for anti-platelet effect
  - Injection morphine sulfate (2–4 mg IV) every 5–10 mins till pain is relieved (max 20 mg total dose)
  - Injection metoclopramide (10 mg IV) to control morphine induced vomiting
  - Injection metoprolol (5 mg IV) every 15 mins (maximum 3 doses); provided pulse rate > 60/min
  - Glyceryl trinitrate by IV infusion pump at a rate of 5 μg/min initially; dose is gradually increased depending on condition of patient
  - Injection streptokinase for reperfusion (only indicated within 6 hours of onset of symptoms)—1.5 million units in 100 mL 0.9% NS by IV infusion over 1 hour
  - Dalteparin sodium (LMWH)—to prevent thromboembolism: 5000 units/12 hours SC injection followed by long term oral warfarin therapy
  - Injection dopamine by continuous IV infusion (if pump failure/shock)—2.5 μg/kg/min and gradually increased till appropriate hemodynamic response
  - If cardiac arrhythmia develops, that should be treated by proper anti-arrhythmic drugs. Use defibrillator if necessary
  - Unless thrombolysis is started within 1-2 hrs of AMI, PCI with stenting is the preferred choice for revascularization whenever available.

6. An overweight middle aged man is found to be hypertensive while attending a clinic for medical cheek up. His BP is 170/105 mm Hg on two successive observations. What will be the treatment for this patient?

MODERATE HYPERTENSION

Presenting Features

Blood pressure—170/105 mm Hg on 2 successive observations.

Relevant Information

The patient is middle aged and overweight.

Inference

The patient is suffering from moderate hypertension which has to be controlled by proper treatment.

Treatment

General Measures

- Moderate salt restriction in diet: Up to 5 gm/day (no added salt)
- Moderate physical exercise and atleast 8 hours of sound sleep every day
- Dietary restriction of calories and fat, weight reduction and consumption of K^+ rich food like banana.
- Stop smoking and restrict alcohol intake

Specific Treatment

- Treatment to be started with monotherapy with:

  Tablet hydrochlorothiazide 25 mg once daily

  Or

  Tablet atenolol 50–100 mg once daily

  Or

  Tablet amlodipine 5–10 mg once daily
- If there is no response, one drug may be combined with another.

7. A 58-year-old man with history of severe hypertension for 20 years, which was well controlled with medication. He stopped taking drugs for a prolonged period. His blood pressure is found to be 240/135 mm Hg with papilledema. What will be the management of this case?

HYPERTENSIVE EMERGENCY

Presenting Features

Blood pressure: 240/135 mm Hg with papilledema.

Relevant Information

A 58-year-old man had history of severe hypertension for 20 years, which was well controlled with medication. Then he stopped taking drugs for a prolonged period.

Inference

This is a case of hypertensive emergency and needs prompt treatment.

Treatment

- The patient is to admitted to ICCU
- Sodium nitroprusside diluted properly in 5% dextrose solution and then administered by controlled continuous IV infusion at a rate of 0.5–1.5 μg/kg/min until blood pressure is reduced to desired level. (30% reduction of pretreatment DBP but not below 95 mm Hg in 1st 48 hours)
- Injection Furosemide 20–40 mg IV may be added to speed up the antihypertensive response.

8. A 25-year-old lady is brought to emergency unit by her family members. She is unconscious with constricted pupils and froth coming out of her mouth. She is reported to consume an organophosphorus insecticide. How will you manage the case?

O-P POISONING

Presenting Features

The patient is unconscious with constricted pupils and froth coming out of her mouth.

Relevant Information

A 25-year-old lady is reported to consume organophosphorus insecticide.

Inference

It is a case of acute organophosphorus compound poisoning.

Treatment

General Supportive Measures

- Removal of contaminated clothing
- Maintenance of airway by aspiration of secretions
- Mechanical ventilation if needed
- IV fluid 5% dextrose-saline infusion
- Diazepam 10 mg IV injection, if there is convulsion.

Specific Treatment

- Atropine sulfate 2–4 mg IV injection. To be repeated every 10 mins until muscarinic symptoms and signs disappear (reduction of salivary and trachea-bronchial secretions, rise in pulse rate, dilatation of pupils). In 1st 24 hours, a maximum of 200 mg of atropine sulfate can be administered
- Pralidoxime chloride 1–2 g IV injection slowly over 5–10 mins. May be repeated after 1 hour if muscle weakness persists (maximum dose is 12 g in 1st 24 hours)
- The patient is observed for 72 hours and atropine sulfate and pralidoxime chloride are to be repeated beyond 24 hours according to the condition of the patient.

9. A middle aged person was watching TV in dark, suddenly develops pain in right eye, vomiting and blurring of vision. On examination, right pupil is dilated, sluggishly reacting to light with raised intraocular pressure. The condition is diagnosed as a case of acute congestive glaucoma. What will be the medical management of this clinical condition?

ACUTE CONGESTIVE GLAUCOMA

Presenting Features

Patient has dilated right pupil, sluggishly reacting to light with raised intraocular pressure.

Relevant Information

A middle aged person while watching TV in dark suddenly developed severe pain in right eye, vomiting and blurring of vision.

Inference

The patient has developed acute congestive glaucoma and needs immediate management.

Treatment

The treatment of choice is surgical, i.e. laser iridotomy/trabeculectomy.

Before surgical intervention, the IOP is to be reduced by drug therapy:
- Hypertonic mannitol 20% solution by IV infusion, 1.5–2 m/kg over a period of 30–60 mins.
- Acetazolamide injection 500 mg IV followed by Acetazolamide tablet 250 mg, 4 times daily
- Pilocarpine nitrate (2% solution), two drops to be instilled in right eye every 10 mins for 1 hour, then at every 30 mins interval till desired IOP is achieved
- Timolol maleate (0.25–0.5% solution), two drops to be instilled in right eye 6 hourly
- Latanoprost (0.005%) or apraclonidine (1%) instillation may be added.

10. A 20-year-old diabetic man on insulin therapy suddenly developed fever and missed his usual doses of insulin and became unconscious. What measures will you take to manage this condition?

MANAGEMENT OF DIABETIC KETOACIDOSIS (DKA)

DKA is a medical emergency and prompt confirmation of diagnosis followed by treatment is of utmost importance.

Principles

- Correcting insulinopenia
- Correct fluid depletion
- Correct dyselectrolytemia
- Treat the underlying etiology or precipitating factor, e.g. infection, infarction, etc.

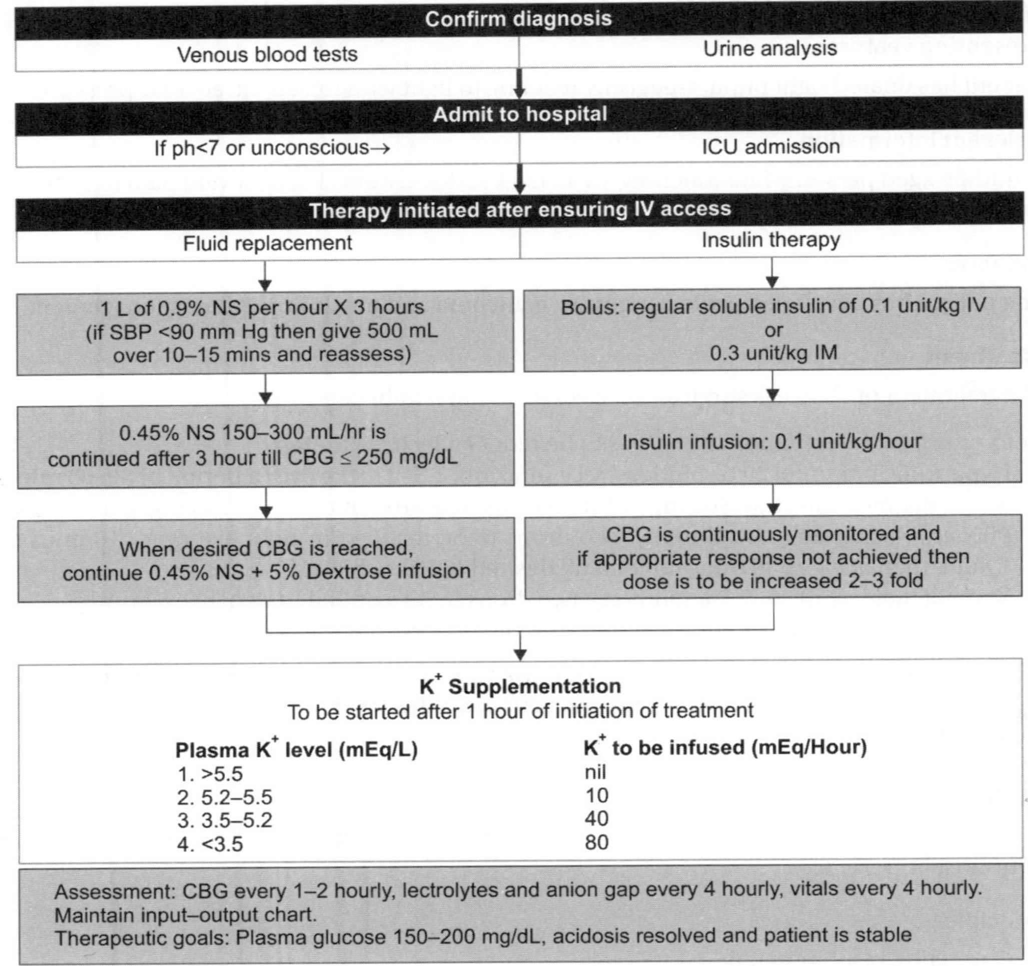

11. A middle-aged diabetic patient with oral anti-diabetic agent (Tolbutamide) underwent prolonged exercise and missed his usual breakfast. He developed unconsciousness, respiratory distress and profuse sweating with tachycardia. How will you manage the case?

HYPOGLYCEMIC COMA

Relevant Information

A middle-aged diabetic patient with oral anti-diabetic agent (Tolbutamide), underwent prolonged exercise and missed his usual breakfast. He developed unconsciousness, respiratory distress and profuse sweating with tachycardia.

Inference

He developed hypoglycemic coma.

Treatment

- IV bolus of 50 mL of 50% dextrose solution followed by continuous IV infusion of 5–10% dextrose solution at a rate of 1–2 mL/min until the patient regains consciousness and is able to take glucose orally
- Injection glucagon 1 mg IM; may be given in severe hypoglycemia and may be repeated after 10 mins if necessary. Effect of glucagon is transient, so it should be supplemented with glucose infusion
- Oral glucose to be initiated once patient is conscious and can tolerate per oral feeds and is to be continued
- Dose of tolbutamide and physical activity should be adjusted to prevent further episodes.

12. A person is willing to travel an endemic area of malaria. What chemoprophylaxis has to be given to him? Subsequently, he developed chloroquine-resistant malaria. How will you manage the case?

CHLOROQUINE-RESISTANT MALARIA

Relevant Information

- A person is willing to travel in an endemic area of malaria
- Even after chemoprophylaxis, he develops chloroquine-resistant malaria.

Inference

- As the person is traveling in an endemic area of malaria, he need chemoprophylaxis.
- When he develops chloroquine-resistant malaria, he needs treatment with proper anti-malarial drugs.

Treatment

- For chemoprophylaxis
  - Tablet chloroquine (300 mg base)—1 tablet weekly (if sensitive)
    To be started 1 week before entering endemic area and continued 4 weeks after leaving it
  - For chloroquine-resistant endemic area:
    Tablet Mefloquine (228 mg base/250 mg base)—1 tablet weekly
    To be started 1 week before entering endemic area and continued 4 weeks after leaving it
  - Alternative to Mefloquine:
    - Tablet Doxycycline hyclate (100 mg)—1 tablet daily
    - To be started 2 days before entering endemic area and continued 4 weeks after leaving it
    - It is to be noted that total duration of therapy shouldn't exceed 4 months.
- For treatment of chloroquine-resistant malaria
  - If patient is conscious
    - Tablet artesunate 100 mg twice daily for 3 days
    - Combined sulfadoxine 500 mg + pyrimethamine 25 mg
    - Tablet- 3 tablets stat on day 1 only
  - If patient is unconscious
    - Injection artesunate 2.4 mg/kg IV at 0, 12 and 24 hours. Then injection artesunate 2.4 mg/kg once daily for 7 days

- Switch over to oral ACT whenever the patient regains consciousness and a full three day course of oral ACT to be given.
- Tablet primaquine 45 mg—1 tablet after clinical cure. The clinical cure is depending upon the species and it coincides with the gametocyte release.

13. A male patient develops fever with chill and rigor. *P. vivax* is found in his blood smear. What will be the management of this case?

Presenting Features

Patient develops fever with chill and rigor.

Relevant Information

P. vivax is found in his blood smear.

Inference

The patient has developed acute attack of vivax malaria.

Treatment

1. Chloroquine phosphate—250 mg (150 mg base)
   Tablet: 4 tablet to be taken immediately followed by 4 tablets after 24 hours and 2 tablets after 24 hours
2. This is followed by primaquine phosphate tablets (50 mg base)—1 tablet daily for 14 days.

14. A woman in 2nd trimester pregnancy is found to be moderately anemic on routine antenatal check-up. What will be the management of this case?

ANEMIA IN PREGNANCY

Presenting Features

A woman is moderately anemic on routine antenatal checkup.

Relevant Information

The woman is in 2nd trimester of pregnancy.

Inference

The woman is suffering from anemia in pregnancy.

Treatment

Ferrous sulfate 200 mg and folic acid 500 μg combined
Tablet—1 tablet 3 times daily after food to be continued till hemoglobin level rises above 10 g%. Then 1 tablet is to be continued for 3 months after delivery.

15. A 6-year-old boy while playing in a village ground was beaten by a snake. The snake was identified as a poisonous one. How will you manage this case?

MANAGEMENT OF SNAKEBITE

Relevant Information

A 6-year-old boy while playing in a village ground was bitten by a poisonous snake.

Inference

It is a case of snakebite poisoning.

Treatment

General Measures

- IV fluids—0.9% Normal saline or 5% dextrose infusion
- Tetanus toxoid (0.5 ml IM injection) and Antibiotic prophylaxis started
- For local pain—paracetamol 650 mg or tramadol 50 mg; repeated every 6–7 hour
- Tramadol 100 mg IV injection for severe pain
- If local swelling spreads, limb should be elevated after administration of antisera
- If there is tourniquet, remove carefully
- Wound is washed with $KMnO_4$ solution

Specific Treatment

- Equine polyvalent antivenom sera (AVS) (against 4 major species available)
- Both liquid and lyophilized form is available in 10 mL vial
- Patient under observation for envenomation.

16. A patient with chronic psychiatric illness was treated with largactil (chlorpromazine) for a prolonged period. He developed tremor, bradykinesia and rigidity. What treatment should be given to the patient without stopping the drug?

DRUG-INDUCED PARKINSONISM

Presenting Features

Patient is having sluggish movements with saliva trickling down the mouth and tremor.

Relevant Information

The patient was attending psychiatry OPD for last 6 months.

Inference

The clinical picture suggests that the patient has developed drug-induced parkinsonism. This is because the commonly prescribed drugs from psychiatry OPD like phenothiazines or Butyrophenones have the propensity to cause extra pyramidal disorders, most commonly Parkinsonism like syndrome.

Treatment

This clinical condition can be managed by administration of anticholinergic drugs. Trihexyphenidyl hydrochloride tablet, 2–12 mg per day in 2–3 divided doses is to be administered. The drug is started with the lowest dose and then gradually uptitrate.

CHAPTER 10

Pharmacy

Avishek Layek, Dyuti Deepta Rano

DEFINITION

Pharmacy is the science that deals with knowledge and art of compounding and dispatching drugs along with their identification, selection, preservation, combination, analysis, and standardization.

PREPARATION OF MAGNESIUM SULFATE PURGATIVE

Compound and Dispense

For Mr X

R_x

- ss Mag sulf 60 mg
- Put two dose marks
- *Direction*: One dose to be taken on the next morning in empty stomach.

Date:____________ ABC

Translation

Symbol	*Latin phrase*	*English phrase*
R_x	Recipe	Take thou, i.e. you take
ss Mag sulf	—	Saturated solution of magnesium sulfate

Ingredients

- Hydrated crystals of magnesium sulfate ($MgSO_4.7H_2O$)
- Water.

Appliances Required

- Simple balance and weight box
- Mortar and pestle
- Mixture phial
- Funnel and cotton
- Pair of scissors
- Piece of paper and gum
- Large measuring cylinder.

Calculations

Solubility of magnesium sulfate at NTP in water is 1:1.5, i.e. 1 g of magnesium sulfate dissolves in 1.5 mL of water producing 2 mL of saturated solution.

So, 1 mL of ss contains 0.5 g of magnesium sulfate
Hence, 60 mL of ss contains 30 g of magnesium sulfate
Similarly, 2 mL of ss contains 1.5 mL of water,
Hence, 60 mL of ss contains 45 mL of water.

Procedure

Preparation of the mixture: 30 g hydrated crystals of magnesium sulfate is measured with simple balance and taken in to the mortar and ground to powder by pestle. 45 mL of water is added by measuring with a large measuring cylinder. The mixture is stirred well until the powder dissolves and then using funnel, it is transferred to mixture phial and corked. Two dose marks are put and the phial is labeled.

Preparation of Label

A piece of paper is cut having a rectangular shape such that it covers the middle third of the body of the phial, with no lateral extension encroaching the border. The label is cut accordingly and borders are drawn around it. Required information is written on it, and it is glued to the surface opposite to the one with the dose mark. The mouth of the phial is corked and it is ready to be dispensed.

THE MIXTURE

No. 1 Date: 28/2/2017

Name : Mr. X

DIRECTION : One dose to be taken next morning in empty stomach.

PHARMACY : NRSMC

SHAKE THE PHIAL BEFORE USE

Sample of a label to be pasted on the body of the phial

Discussion

1. Define mixture.

Mixture is a liquid preparation containing medical ingredients, usually dispensed in several doses meant for oral administration for local, systemic as well as reflex actions, e.g. sodium bicarbonate acting as expectorant by reflex action.

2. What are the types of mixtures?

- *Simple mixture*: Containing soluble ingredients
- *Compound mixture*:
  - Mixtures containing insoluble but diffusible solids, e.g. magnesium trisilicate
  - Mixtures containing insoluble and indiffusible solid. They require a suspending agent, e.g. Creta (chalk).

3. What is saturated solution?

It is a solution containing maximum amount of the solute in the dissolved state at a particular temperature and pressure.

4. What is the strength of ss magnesium sulfate?

25% (hypertonic).

5. What is a super saturated solution?

A solution containing an additional amount of solute in dissolved state in an already saturated solution by raising temperature or pressure or both. By lowering the temperature or pressure or both, the solute will precipitate.

6. What are the actions of magnesium sulfate?

- *Locally*: Reduction of swelling and pain of inflammation (antiphlogistic action)
- *Orally*: Saline purgative
- *Rectally*: As retention enema to reduce raised intra cranial tension (ICT)
- *Parenterally*: Anticonvulsant as intramuscular (IM) and tocolytic effect on intravenous (IV).

7. Contraindications of magnesium sulfate?

- Pregnancy (but used in preeclampsia)
- Renal insufficiency
- Piles
- Organic intestinal obstruction
- Appendicitis
- Undiagnosed abdominal pain.

8. What are the adverse effects of prolonged purgative use?

- Loss of water and electrolytes
- Deficiency of calories, minerals and vitamins due to interference in absorption
- Spastic colitis
- Dyspepsia
- Anorexia
- Nausea
- Loss of normal rectal reflex
- Dependency.

9. What is the antidote of ss magnesium sulfate?

Intravenous calcium gluconate.

PREPARATION OF CARMINATIVE MIXTURE

Compound and Dispense

For Mr X

R_x

- Sodi. bicarb 1 g
- Comp tinct card 2 mL
- Arom Sp of ammon 1 mL
- Water added up to 30 mL
- Mix and make one dose of mixture
- Send two such doses
- *Direction*: One dose to be taken twice daily after meals.

Date:________ ABC

Translation

Symbol	*Latin phrase*	*English phrase*
R_x	recipe	take thou, i.e. you take
Sodi bicarb	–	Sodium bicarbonate
Comp tinct card	–	compound tincture of cardamom
Arom Sp of ammon	–	aromatic spirit of ammonia

Ingredients

- Sodium bicarbonate
- Compound tincture of cardamom
- Aromatic spirit of ammonia
- Water.

Appliances Required

- Simple balance and weight box
- Mortar and pestle
- Mixture phial
- Funnel and cotton
- Pair of scissors
- Piece of paper and gum
- Large and small measuring cylinder
- Glass stirrer.

Calculation

Required amount of respective ingredients for preparation of two doses are as follows:

- Sodium bicarbonate: 1 × 2 = 2 g
- Compound tincture of cardamom: 2 × 2 = 4 mL
- Aromatic spirit of ammonia: 1 × 2 = 2 mL
- Water: Up to 60 mL.

Procedure

Preparation of the Dose Marking

60 mL of water is measured with a large measuring cylinder and taken in the mixture phial. A strip of paper measuring 0.5 inch thick is taken with its upper margin coinciding with the lower meniscus of the water column and the lower margin coinciding with the midpoint between the flat and curved part of the base of the phial. The paper is folded on itself to make two equal halves and indentations are cut on the two ends of the midline and also four corners to the strip to give a shape of an octagon over another. 60 mL of water is then discarded.

Preparation of Mixture Proper

2 g of sodium bicarbonate is taken after measuring with simple balance and is firmly ground with mortar and pestle. 45 mL of water is measured with the help of a large measuring cylinder and transferred to the mortal and mixed well with glass stirrer. Then 4 mL of the compound cardamom tincture is measured with small measuring cylinder and added to mixture. The mixture is transferred to the phial with the help of a funnel. Then 2 mL of aromatic spirit of ammonia is measured with small measuring cylinder and added to mixture phial. Finally, water is added up to 60 mL, such that the upper level of dose marking and upper level of mixture coincide.

Preparation of Label

A piece of paper is cut in a rectangular shape such that it covers the middle third of the body of the phial, with no lateral extension encroaching the border. The label is cut accordingly and borders are drawn around it. Required information is written on it and it is glued to the surface opposite to the one with the dose mark. The mouth of the phial is corked and it is ready to be dispensed.

THE MIXTURE

No. 2 Date: 17/3/17

Name: Mr. X

Direction: One dose to be taken twice daily after meals

PHARMACY – NRSMC

SHAKE THE PHIAL BEFORE USE

Sample of label

Discussion

10. What are carminatives?

Carminatives are drugs which cause expulsion of gases from within stomach and intestinal lumen.

11. What are the carminative principles present in thus mixture?

- Sodium bicarbonate
- Volatile oils and other ingredients of compound cardamom tincture and aromatic spirit of ammonia.

12. What is tincture?

An alcoholic solution of crude vegetable drugs obtained by percolation or maceration.

13. What is the composition of tincture of cardamom?

- Caraway oil
- Cardamom oil
- Cinnamon oil
- Glycerin
- Alcohol
- Cochineal/Amaranth plant product
- Coloring agent: *Cochineal*—it is the dried female insect called *Coccus cacti* or Spanish fly (*Dactylopius cocci*).

14. What is spirit?

Alcoholic solution/preparation of a volatile substance.

15. What is composition of aromatic spirit of ammonia?

- Ammonium bicarbonate
- Strong solution of ammonia
- Oil of lemon
- Alcohol
- Oil of nutmeg
- Distilled water.

16. How does sodium bicarbonate act as carminative?

- $NaHCO_3 + HCl = NaCl + H_2O + CO_2$ [source of HCl is stomach]
- Evolved CO_2 is responsible for carminative effect.

17. How volatile oils act as carminative?

They cause mild irritation and thus increase GI motility and cause sphincter relaxation; thereby helping in gas expulsion.

18. What are the uses of carminative mixture?

It is used to relieve flatulence and also gas colics in the absence of a definite mechanical obstruction:

- In infants and children, aerophagia
- Defective absorption of gases as in CCF, portal cirrhosis, etc.

- Indigestion
- Aerophagia in psychoneurotic adults.

19. Name some modern carminatives.

- *Methyl polysiloxane*: Defoaming agent
- *Simethicone*: Surface lowering agent.

PREPARATION OF CALAMINE LOTION

Compound and Dispense

For Mr. X

R_x

- Calamine 15 g
- Zinc oxide 5 g
- Bentonite 3 g
- Sodium citrate 0.5 g
- Liquefied phenol 0.5 mL
- Glycerin 5 mL
- Purified water added up to 100 mL
- Mix and make a lotion
- *Direction*: To be applied locally twice daily.

Date:____________ ABC

Translation

Symbol	*Latin phrase*	*English phrase*
R_x	Recipe	Take thou, i.e you take

Ingredients

- Calamine
- Zinc oxide
- Bentonite
- Sodium citrate
- Liquefied phenol
- Glycerin
- Purified water.

Appliances Required

- Simple balance and weight box
- Mortar and pestle
- Lotion bottle
- Funnel and cotton
- Pair of scissors
- Piece of paper and gum
- Large and small measuring cylinder.

Calculations

For 100 mL of calamine lotion, we use the following ingredients in the respective quantities:

- Calamine 15 g
- Zinc oxide 5 g
- Bentonite 3 g
- Sodium citrate 0.5 g
- Liquefied phenol 0.5 mL
- Glycerin 5 mL
- Purified water added up to 100 mL.

Procedure

Preparation of Lotion

With the help of simple balance and weights, measure 0.5 g sodium citrate and take in to the mortar. It is then powdered finely by pestle. Calamine 15 g, zinc oxide 5 g, and bentonite 3 g are measured and added to the mortar, and mixed well and powdered by pestle. Now, 30 mL of purified water is measured with large measuring cylinder and poured into the mortal to mix it well. Now, with the small measuring cylinder, 0.5 mL liquid phenol and 5 mL glycerin is added in the mortar and mixed well. With the help of funnel, this is transferred to large measuring cylinder and purified water is added to make the lotion up to 100 mL. Lotion is then poured in to the lotion bottle. Then the lotion bottle is corked and labeling is done.

Preparation of Label

A rectangular piece of paper having the length of one-third of that of the bottle and breadth little less than half the circumference with all relevant information written on it is taken. Borders are drawn and then this paper is pasted on the middle one-third of the bottle. The lotion is now ready to dispense.

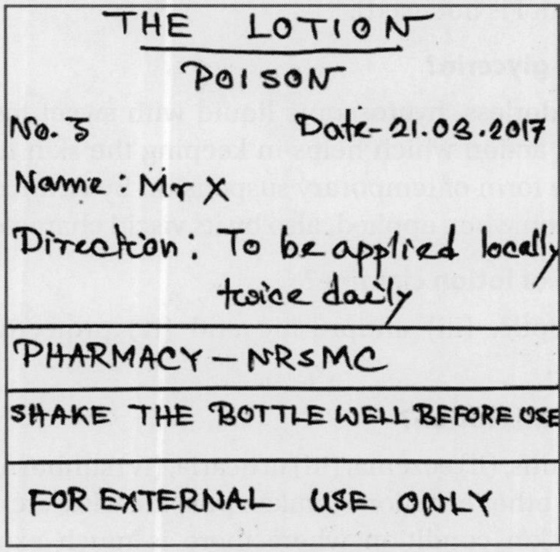

Sample of label for lotion

Discussion

20. Is this an official lotion?

It is the only official lotion as advocated by Indian Pharmacopeia. Other lotions are extemporaneous.

21. What is lotion?

It is a thick, smooth liquid based preparation designed to be applied to the skin for medicinal or cosmetic purposes.

22. What is calamine?

It is a mild astringent, antiseptic and protective. Chemically, it is basic zinc carbonate 98% colored with 2% ferric oxide (gives pink color).

23. What is bentonite?

It is an adsorbent and suspending agent used for insoluble powders in the lotion. Chemically, it is native colloidal hydrated aluminum silicate (free from grittiness).

24. What are the actions of zinc oxide?

It has mild astringent, soothing and protective effects on skin.

25. What is the function of sodium citrate?

As it is highly water soluble, sodium citrate acts a suspending agent by decreasing viscosity produced by bentonite and converts the gel to sol.

26. What is liquefied phenol?

Phenol in liquid form which contains 80% of phenol (w/v) (100 mL of liquefied phenol contains 80 g of phenol in distilled water). 0.5% strength—exerts local anesthetic effect and so acts as antipruritic agent and has weak antiseptic action.
(Solid phenol is hygroscopic; it draws water from atmosphere and standard cannot be maintained. So, solid phenol is not used).

27. What is the action of glycerin?

Glycerin is a colorless, odorless, hygroscopic liquid with sweet taste. It is soluble in water (1:3). It exerts demulcent action which helps in keeping the skin moist and soft; also keeps the insoluble solids in the form of temporary suspension by virtue of its viscid character and prevents drying of the lotion when applied, also by its viscid character.

28. What are the actions of lotion clamine?

(i) Astringent, (ii) antiseptic, (iii) antipruritic and (iv) protective; so sometimes called astringent, sedative lotion.

29. What are the uses of this lotion?

(i) Acute exudative dermatitis, (ii) eczema, (iii) urticaria, (iv) sunburn, (v) bed sores, (vi) napkin rash, and (vii) herpes and other eruptions (chiken pox, measles, etc).
It is contraindicated in skin condition where there is much exudation because of crust formation.

PREPARATION OF GAMMA BENZENE HEXACHLORIDE OINTMENT

Compound and Dispense

For Mr X

R_x

- Gamma benzene hexachloride powder 100 mg
- Yellow soft paraffin 9.9 g
- Mix and make an ointment
- Direction: To be applied from neck to feet by gentle rubbing.

Date:__________ ABC

Translation

Symbol	*Latin phrase*	*English phrase*
R_x	Recipe	Take thou, i.e. you take

Ingredients

- Gamma benzene hexachloride powder
- Yellow soft paraffin.

Appliances Required

- Simple balance and weight box
- Pill tile
- Ointment pot (Galli's)
- Pair of spatula
- Pair of scissors
- Piece of white paper and oil paper
- Rubber band
- Glue.

Calculation

- 10 g of ointment contains 100 mg of gamma benzene hexachloride.
- So, 1 g of ointment contains 10 mg of gamma benzene hexachloride.
- Hence, 100 g of ointment contains 1,000 mg or 1g of gamma benzene hexachloride.
- Hence, the strength of the ointment is 1%.

Procedure

Preparation of the Ointment Proper

100 mg of gamma benzene hexachloride and 9.9 g of yellow soft paraffin are weighted separately with a simple balance and weights. The powder is placed at the center of the pill tile while the yellow soft paraffin at one of its four corners (in order to minimize the wastage of the drug powder due to displacement of fanning out). A small amount of the paraffin is drawn toward the center of the pill tile and thoroughly mixed with a small amount of powder by circular motion of one spatula. The same process is repeated several times, until all the amount of

powder is thoroughly mixed with paraffin to yield a homogeneous smooth nongritty and pasty appearance of the whole material.

Preparation of Circular Label

A circular flap of white paper is drawn by keeping the ointment pot upside down on the piece of white paper and adhering the point of a pen to the circumferential rim at the mouth top the pot. This flap is cut out from the rest of the paper and necessary information is duly written on it.

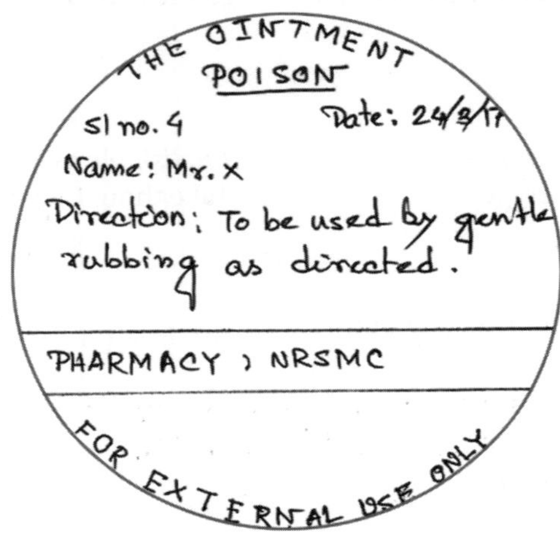

Sample of circular label

With the help of the two spatulas simultaneously, the ointment is now transferred into the Galli's pot—one spatula is used to hold the material, while the other to scrape it off in to the pot. Care is taken in this process, so that the whole mass falls down to the center the floor of the pot and no part of it sticks to the wall of the pot.

The mouth of the pot is finally closed with a piece of oil-paper and fixed in situ with a rubber band. Finally, the circular label made of white paper is pasted on the upper surface of the oil paper. The preparation is now ready to dispense.

Discussion

30. What is an ointment?

It is a soft or semisolid preparation containing medicinal ingredients in a suitable basis for external application.

31. What are the uses of this ointment?

Scabies: a parasitic infestation of a female mite, *Acarus scabiei* (Sarcoptes scabiei).

32. How to apply this ointment in scabies?

After a hot scrubbing soap bath, the ointment is applied from neck to feet except scalp and face and kept overnight. Next morning, a warm soap bath is to be taken with thorough cleaning of garments worn at night and bed linen.

33. What are the other drugs used in scabies?

- 25% emulsion of benzyl benzoate
- Permethrin
- *Ivermectin*: only oral drug available for scabies
- 1% sulfur ointment
- Crotamiton
- Monosulfiram
- Thiabendazole.

34. Does the dose need repetition?

Yes, may be repeated after a week.

35. What are the side effects?

Neurotoxicity, hematotoxicity and mutagenicity.

36. What are the contraindications?

Pregnancy and premature infants.

PREPARATION OF ATROPINE SULFATE EYE OINTMENT

Compound and Dispense

For Mr X

R_x

- Atropine sulfate powder 100 mg
- Yellow soft paraffin 9.9 g
- Mix and make an ointment
- Direction: To be applied on lower eyelid margin, twice daily.

Date:____________ ABC

Translation:

Symbol	*Latin phrase*	*English phrase*
R_x	Recipe	Take thou, i.e. you take

Ingredients

- Atropine sulfate powder
- Yellow soft paraffin.

Appliances Required

- Simple balance and weight box
- Pill tile
- Ointment pot (Galli's)
- Pair of spatula
- Pair of scissors
- Piece of white paper and oil paper
- Rubber band
- Glue.

Calculation

- 10 g of ointment contains 100 mg of atropine sulfate
- So, 1 g of ointment contains 10 mg of atropine sulfate
- Hence, 100 g of ointment contains 1,000 mg or 1g of atropine sulfate.
- Hence, the strength of the ointment is 1%.

Procedure

Preparation of the Ointment Proper

100 mg of atropine sulfate and 9.9 g of yellow soft paraffin are weighted separately with a simple balance and weights. The powder is placed at the center of the pill tile while the yellow soft paraffin at one of its four corners (in order to minimize the wastage of the drug powder due to displacement of fanning out). A small amount of the paraffin is drawn toward the center of the pill tile and thoroughly mixed with a small amount of powder by circular motion of one spatula. The same process is repeated several times, until all the amount of powder are thoroughly mixed with paraffin to yield a homogeneous smooth non gritty and pasty appearance of the whole material.

Preparation of Circular Label

A circular flap of white paper is drawn by keeping the ointment pot upside down on the piece of white paper and adhering the point of a pen to the circumferential rim at the mouth top the pot. This flap is cut out from the rest of the paper and necessary information is duly written on it.

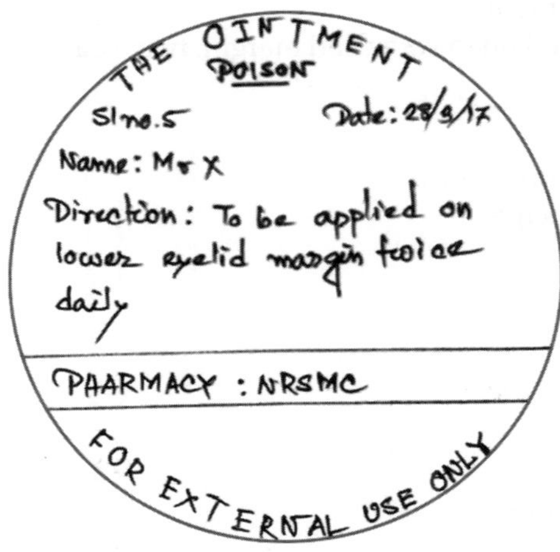

Other sample of circular label

With the help of the two spatulas simultaneously, the ointment is now transferred into the Galli's pot—one spatula is used to hold the material, while the other to scrape it off in to the pot. Care is taken in this process, so that the whole mass falls down to the center the floor of the pot and no part of it sticks to the wall of the pot.

The mouth of the pot is finally closed with a piece of oil-paper and fixed in situ with a rubber band. Finally, the circular label made of white paper is pasted on the upper surface of the oil paper. The preparation is now ready to dispense.

Discussion

37. How to apply?

Lower eyelid margins to be everted and then to apply on the eylid margins.

38. Why yellow soft paraffin but not white soft paraffin is used?

White soft paraffin is prepared by bleaching of yellow soft paraffin with chlorine; so, this chlorine may cause irritation of the eye.

39. What are the effects of this ointment on eye?

- Mydriasis—passive dilatation of pupil as the muscarinic effect on constrictor pupillae is blocked and unopposed effect of sympathetic dialatory fibres (alpha effect) occurs.
- Cycloplegia (paralysis of accommodation)—Paralysis of ciliary muscle → suspensory ligament of lens are taught → lens are prevented from being more convex, i.e. flattening of lens → Paralysis of accomodation → Eye is fiex for distant vision and near objects are blurred.
- Loss of light reflex—As the constrictor pupillae cannot function
- Intraocular tension (normal 12–20 mm Hg) may rise and may precipitate glaucoma. Narrowing of iridocorneal angle and thus prevention of drainage of aqueous humor through the canal of Schlemm situated at the iridocorneal angle.
- Drying of the conjunctiva due to inhibition of lacrimal secretion
- Paradoxical circumcorneal hyperemia/congestion due to dilatation of conjunctival blood vessels.
- Photophobia due to pupillary dilation.

40. What are the sources of atropine?

Atropine is an alkaloid, obtained from *Atropa belladonna, Datura stramonium, Hyoscyamus niger-all parts.*

41. What are the uses of this ointment?

- As a mydriatic and cycloplegic for accurate measurement of errors of refraction in children below the age of 5 years (because in children parasympathetic tone is high). For children over 5 years and in adults, cyclopentolate (0.5%) Or tropicamide (0.5%) or homatropine hydrobromide (2%) is used and this helps to determine the far point of eye easily. Mydriasis is often necessary for thorough examination of the retina and optic disk. Cyclopentolate and tropicamide lack cycloplegic effect.
- In the treatment of acute iritis where the above mydriatics act by two ways:
  - Prolonged mydriasis causes prolonged relaxation of iris.
  - Patient abandons his efforts of accommodation because he realises that he cannot focus for near vision. So, iris will get rest. Any of the above mydriatics is instilled as 2 drops 3 times a day.
- In treatment of iridocyclitis, choroiditis, following cataract extraction, keratitis, complete cycloplegia and mydriasis are required in thiese conditions and it is instilled as 2 drops 3 times a day.

- In treatment of posterior synechiae, tropine may be alternated with miotics to prevent or break adhesions between the iris and the lens.

42. What are the contraindications of use of atropine ointment in eye?

- Norrow-angle glaucoma/chronic wide angle glaucoma
- Intraocular lens transplantation
- Subluxated lens
- History of hypersensitivity to atropine (local irritation of eye, may produced swelling of the eyelids and conjunctivitis).

43. How long the effects of atropine remain?

About 7–10 days, if not counteracted by cholinergic drugs. Only partially counteracted by pilocarpine (2%), physostigmine (0.5%) or DFP (0.025%).

44. How will you differentiate mydriasis produced by sympathomimetic agent (ephedrine, phenylephrine) from the same caused by muscarinic blockers?

- Light reflex lost in atropine-induced mydriasis but not in mydriasis produced by sympathomimetic agent, because the pupillae remains intact and can be tested both in animals and human beings.
- Loss of accommodation observed in atropine-induced mydriasis but not in sympathomimetic induced mydriasis as there is cycloplegia and can be tested in human beings only.
- Conjunctival congestion is observed in atropine-induced mydriasis but blanching of conjunctiva is observed in sympathomimetic agent-induced mydriasis. This can be observed from distance.

45. What are the uses of atropine?

- As antisecretory
  - Preanesthetic medication
  - Peptic ulcer
  - Pulmonary embolism
- As antispasmodic
  - Intestinal colic, renal colic and abdominal cramps; in absence of mechanical obstruction
  - Nervous, functional and drug induced diarrhea
  - Spastic constipation
  - Irritable bowel syndrome
  - Pylorospasm
  - Gastric hypermotility
  - Gastritis, nervous dyspepsia
  - To relieve urinary frequency and urgency
  - Dysmenorrhea
- Bronchial asthma, asthmatic bronchitis, COPD
- As mydriatic and cycloplegic
- As cardiac vagolytic
  - Sinus bradycardia
  - Partial heart block
- For central action
  - Parkinsonism
  - Motion sickness

- To antagonize muscarinic effects of drugs and poisons
  - Organophosphates (OPs) poisoning
  - Early mushroom poisoning.

46. What are the side effects of atropine?

- Dry mouth, difficulty in swallowing and speech
- Dry flushed and hot skin, fever
- Difficulty in micturition
- Dilated pupil causing photophobia and blurring of near vision
- Palpitation
- Excitement, psychotic behavior, ataxia, delirium, dreadful visual hallucinations
- Hypotension, weak and rapid pulse, cardiovascular collapse
- Respiratory depressions.
- Convulsion or coma in severe poisoning—"hot as a hare, blind as a bat, dry as a bone, red as a beet and mad as a hatter

PREPARATION OF ORAL REHYDRATION SALT POWDER

Compound and Dispense

For Mr X

R_x

- Sodium chloride 2.6 g
- Trisodium citrate dehydrate 2.9 g
- Potassium chloride 1.5 g
- Glucose 13.5 g
- Mix and make a powder
- Direction: The whole powder is to be dissolved in one liter of safe drinking water and to drink as directed.

Date:____________ ABC

Translation:

Symbol	*Latin phrase*	*English phrase*
R_x	Recipe	Take thou, i.e. you take

- Ingredients
  - Sodium chloride
  - Trisodium citrate dehydrate
  - Potassium chloride
  - Glucose.
- Appliances
  - Simple balance and weight box
  - Mortar and pestle
  - Envelope
  - Pair of scissors
  - Piece of white paper and oil paper
  - Glue.

Calculation

Required amounts of ingredients are:

- Sodium chloride 2.6 g
- Trisodium citrate dehydrate 2.9 g
- Potassium chloride 1.5 g
- Glucose 13.5 g.

Procedure

Preparation of Powder Proper

Sodium chloride 2.6 g, trisodium citrate dehydrate 2.9 g, potassium chloride 1.5 g and glucose 13.5 g are weighed using simple balance and taken in to the mortar.

They are ground and mixed with the help of pestle to make a powder. The powder is then transferred into an envelope and the envelope is then sealed with a glue.

Preparation of Label

A white paper is cut to size in such a way that a uniform gap of 0.5 cm remains all around between the respective border of the envelope and the label. A margin is drawn all around the label and after writing all the information, it is pasted on the envelope using glue. The powder is then ready to dispense.

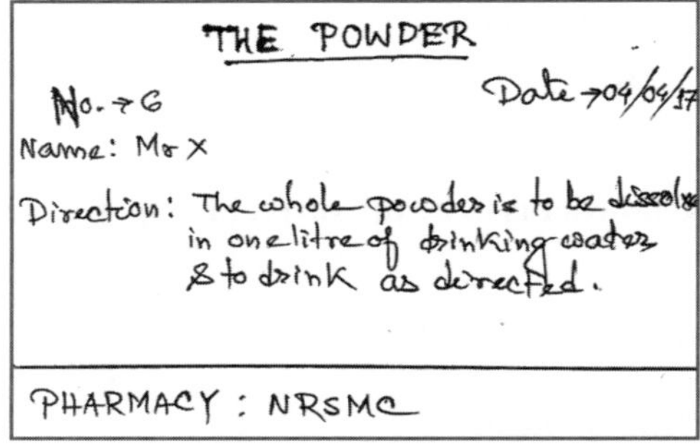

Other example of label

Discussion

47. What is the composition of ORS?

As described in the prescription.

48. What was the original WHO formula?

In original formula, $NaHCO_3$ (2.5 g) was given in place of sodium citrate (2.9 g); other ingredients remaining the same.

49. Why $NaHCO_3$ was replaced by sodium citrate?

ORS, on keeping becomes caked and develops a brown colour due to formation of furfural compounds by chemical reaction between $NaHCO_3$ and glucose. Replacement of $NaHCO_3$ by sodium citrate makes the preparation more stable, because sodium citrate has a longer shelf-life and does not undergo this reaction.

50. What are the general principles followed during formulation of ORS?

- 'ORS should be isotonic (because diarrhea fluids are approx. isotonic with plasma).
- The molar conc. of glucose should be somewhat higher that Na^+ present in the intestinal secretions in addition to that present in ORS itself.
- Sufficient amount of K^+ and HCO^-_3 must be present to make up the losses in the stool.

51. On what basis the composition of ORS is formulated?

The composition of ORS is based on the composition of cholera stools, particularly in children.

52. What are the common causes of infective diarrhea?

There are three important causes of infective diarrhea: (a) Cholera, (b) Enterobacteria (*Shigella*, enteropathogenic *E. coli*, *Salmonella*, etc.) and *E. histolytica* (common in developing countries), and (c) Retrovirus (common in developed countries).

Note: In type-II infective diarrhea, Na^+ loss in stool is less than cholera stools. So, during treatment with ORS, there is chance of hypernatremia, particularly in children (manifested as puffiness of eylid). Mother is advised to administer ORS and plain water in 2:1 ratio to avoid this hypernatremia.

53. How does ORS produced beneficial effect in diarrhea?

ORS replaces the fluid and electrolytes lost in diarrhea and thus helps to maintain the fluid and electrolyte balance.

- Glucose helps in the transport of sodium and water across the intestinal epithelium (facilitated diffusion).
- K^+ replaces the K^+ loss in diarrhea.
- Citrate/bicarbonate corrects acidosis (HCO^-_3 is lost in diarrhea leading to acidosis). It may also promote Na^+ and water reabsorption.

54. What happens if higher conc. of glucose is added?

Higher conc. of glucose increases the risk of osmotic diarrhea and dehydration is increased. So, glucose more than 20 g/L should never be used.
Note: Sucrose (40 g) can be used as a substitute of glucose. It is slowly acting.

55. What are the indications of ORS?

- Mild diarrhea (fluid loss is 7.5–10% of body weight)
- Moderate diarrhea (fluid loss is 7.5–10% of body weight
- Maintenance therapy of severe diarrhea after rehydration by IV fluids.
- Nondiarrheal uses—(i) postsurgical, postburn, posttrauma maintenance of hydration and nutrition, (ii) heart stroke and (iii) during changeover from parenteral to enteral administration.

56. How to administer ORS?

- In the initial stage of therapy:
  i. Mild diarrhea—50 mL/kg within 4 hours
  ii. Moderate diarrhea—100 mL/kg within 4 hours

- Maintenance therapy—The general principles is that the oral fluid intake should be equal to the continuing stool loss. Adults and older children are advised to drink as much as they want to satisfy their thirst. Roughly 100 mL/kg/day until diarrhea stops is required in mild cases. For severe diarrhea, it is 10–15 mL/kg/hour.

57. Any special advice is to be given to the mother?

- If child is breat fed, continue breastfeeding.
- If the child is not breast fed, ORS and plain water are to be given in 2:1 ratio (To avoid puffiness of the eyelid due to hypernatremia).
- If puffiness of the eyelids develops, stop ORS, continue plain water or breast milk till puffiness
- If the child vomits, wait for 10 min and then continue ORS, but more slowly.
- Food normally taken by the child should be continued
- The solution once prepared, should be used up within 12–24 hours to avoid bacterial contamination. Solution should not be boiled or sterilized.

58. What are the indications of IV rehydration?

- Severe dehydration
- Patient in shock
- Patients unable to drink.

59. Name the solutions used for IV rehydration?

- Ringer lactate solution supplying sufficient amount of sodium, potassium and lactate yielding bicarbonate.
- Diarrhea treatment solution (DTS) containing sodium chloride (4 g), sodium acetate (6.5 g), potassium chloride (1 g) and glucose (10 g).
- Normal saline is often used, but it does not correct acidosis and will not replace potasium loss; it is the poorest fluid.

Note: 5% dextrose solution is better to be avoided because it only provides water and glucose but no electrolytes and acidosis is not corrected.

60. What is the composition of "home recipe" ORS/L?

Table salt	3/4 tablespoon
Baking soda	1 teaspoon
Orange juice	1 cup
Table sugar	4 level tablespoon

Food-based oral rehydration formulations prepared by replacing table sugar with 50–60 g of cereal flour or 200 g of mashed boiled potato, may help to reduce fluid output.

61. What is rice based oral rehydration salt solution?

To prepare a rice based ORS solution, 50 g of rice powder replacing 20 g of glucose should be boiled in 1.1L of water for about 8 min, should be cooled, and then salts as recommended for the WHO—ORS solution should be added and mixed well before being served. Rice based ORS solution should be used within 6-8 hours.

CHAPTER 11

Drug Interaction

Arnab Pal

AMOXICILLIN AND CLAVULANIC ACID

Type

It is a pharmacokinetic type of drug interaction.

Result of Interaction

Amoxicillin becomes more effective against penicillinase/beta-lactamase producing organisms like staphylococci, gonococci, etc.

Mechanism of Interaction

Amoxicillin is an extended spectrum beta-lactam aminopenicillin. Clavulanic acid is a beta-lactamase inhibitor obtained from *Streptomyces clavuligerus.* The antibacterial action of amoxicillin is due to presence of beta-lactam ring which is broken by beta-lactamase produced by certain microbes. Clavulanic acid acts as a suicide inhibitor and the beta-lactam ring in its compound binds to the beta-lactamases, thus inactivating them. Decrease in beta-lactamase action thus promotes penicillin action.

Remarks

Cotherapy of these two benefits the patient. Fixed-dose combination (FDC) of amoxicillin 250 mg + clavulanic acid 125 mg is used.

METRONIDAZOLE AND ETHYL ALCOHOL

Type

This is an example of pharmacokinetic type of drug interaction.

Result of Interaction

Chance of precipitation of "antabuse" (disulfiram-like) reaction characterized by nausea, vomiting, abdominal cramps, and hypotension.

Mechanism of Interaction

Metronidazole is a nitroimidazole used to treat many bacterial and protozoal infections. Ethyl alcohol is a commonly used beverage. Ethyl alcohol is metabolized in two steps—first converted to acetaldehyde and then to acetic acid by dehydrogenases. Acetic acid is released from our body in the form of CO_2 and H_2O. Metronidazole inhibits the second step, i.e. aldehyde dehydrogenase leading to accumulation of acetaldehyde in our system. This leads to the above-mentioned clinical features.

Remarks

These two should not be coadministered. If a nitroimidazole is at all to be used secnidazole or satranidazole may be used.

CIPROFLOXACIN AND THEOPHYLLINE

Type

It is a pharmacokinetic type of drug interaction at the level of drug metabolism.

Result of Interaction

Increased side effects of theophylline, such as palpitation, hypotension, cardiac arrhythmias, and convulsion may occur.

Mechanism of Interaction

Ciprofloxacin is one of the most commonly used fluoroquinolone bactericidal antibiotic. Theophylline is a methylxanthine used in asthma. The major pathway of theophylline metabolism involves 8-hydroxylation resulting in formation and excretion of 1,3-desmethyl uric acid. Ciprofloxacin inhibits the metabolism of theophylline by inhibition of 8-hydroxylation pathway and increases concentration of theophylline beyond therapeutic level.

Plasma Concentration of Theophylline

- *Therapeutic level*: 10–15 μg/mL
- Side effects as mentioned earlier other than seizures occur at 20 μg/mL
- Seizures occur at 30–40 μg/mL.

Remarks

Coadministration of both these drugs should be avoided.

ASPIRIN AND WARFARIN

Type

It is an example of both pharmacodynamics as well as pharmacokinetic drug interaction.

Result of Interaction

Increased bleeding tendency from various sites.

Mechanism of Interaction

Aspirin is a prototype example of nonsteroidal anti-inflammatory drug (NSAID). Warfarin sodium is an *in vivo* acting and mostly used oral anticoagulant.

- *Pharmacodynamic*: Warfarin sodium increases prothrombin time by inhibiting the synthesis of vitamin K-dependent coagulation factors (II, VII, IX, and X). Aspirin increases bleeding time and interferes in the normal hemostasis by inhibiting platelet aggregation due to disbalance between $PGI_2$and TXA_2. Moreover, aspirin is ulcerogenic in stomach and duodenum.
- *Pharmacokinetic*: Aspirin may displace warfarin from plasma protein binding site that act as silent receptors, resulting in increased levels of free warfarin in plasma.

Remarks

It is better to avoid this combination, if all the antiplatelets are to be given along with warfarin; dipyridamole/ticlopidine may be used.

RIFAMPICIN AND COMBINED ORAL CONTRACEPTIVE PILL

Type

It is a pharmacokinetic type of drug interaction at the level of drug metabolism.

Result of Interaction

Failure of contraception and menstrual irregularities in the form of spotting/breakthrough bleeding.

Mechanism of Interaction

Rifampicin is a semisynthetic, bactericidal agent effective against mycobacterial infections. Combined oral contraceptive pill (OCP) is an example of FDC of ethinyl estradiol and norethindrone acetate. Rifampicin is a hepatic microsomal enzyme inducer including CYP 3A4, CYP 2D6, CYP 1A2, and CYP 2C subfamily. The same enzymes also metabolize estrogen and progesterone components of the OCP and hence there may be fall of therapeutic concentration and failure of contraception results.

Remarks

The patient should be asked to take higher dose of OCP or should be advised other methods of contraception ex-intrauterine device.

CHLOROQUINE AND ALKALI MIXTURE

Type

It is a pharmacokinetic type of drug interaction at the level of renal excretion.

Result of Interaction

Increased side effects of chloroquine such as hypotension, vasodilation, suppressed myocardial function, electrocardiogram changes, cardiac arrest, visual disturbances, headache, and lichenoid skin eruptions.

Mechanism of Interaction

Chloroquine is an antimalarial drug. Alkali mixture is a commonly used mixture in fever to counteract pyrexia induced actions. Chloroquine is a basic drug. It is usually excreted in urine in unchanged fraction (>50%) and as its metabolite monodesethyl chloroquine (~20%). Alkali mixture may raise the urinary pH, so there is less ionization of chloroquine and major portion of chloroquine present in tubular fluid remains unionized. This unionized chloroquine will be reabsorbed and plasma concentration will rise above therapeutic concentration.

Remarks

These two drugs should not be coadministered.

SUCRALFATE AND ANTACID

Type

It is a pharmacodynamic type of drug interaction.

Result of Interaction

The cytoprotective effect of sucralfate on gastrointestinal mucosa is reduced.

Mechanism of Interaction

Antacids are drugs which neutralize the gastric HCl by chemical action and raise pH of gastric contents. Sucralfate is an ulcer protective agent which strongly adheres to the base of ulcer and thereby protects it from peptic digestion. Sucralfate complex is formed by sucral octasulfate and polyaluminum hydroxide. In pH less than 4, the complex undergoes extensive polymerization and cross linking to form a sticky viscid yellow white gel which adheres to the ulcer base for more than 6 hours. Antacids by raising gastric pH prevent polymerization and thereby reduce the ulcer protective effect.

Remarks

These two drugs should not be administered simultaneously. If at all used, sucralfate is to be used 30 minutes after antacid ingestion.

L-DOPA AND PYRIDOXINE

Type

It is a pharmacodynamic type of drug interaction at the level of decarboxylation of L-DOPA.

Result of Interaction

The availability of dopamine in the central nervous system (CNS) is reduced, hence the anti-parkinsonism effect of L-DOPA is reduced.

Mechanism of Interaction

L-DOPA is used in the treatment of idiopathic Parkinsonism. Pyridoxine is vitamin B_6 and acts a cofactor of DOPA-decarboxylase enzyme. Peripheral conversion of L-DOPA to dopamine by DOPA-decarboxylase is enhanced by pyridoxine and consequently the availability of dopamine in basal ganglia of CNS is reduced as only L-DOPA and not dopamine can cross blood–brain barrier. Thus beneficial effect of L-DOPA in Parkinsonism is reduced.

Remarks

These two drugs should not be coadministered.

PROPRANOLOL AND VERAPAMIL

Type

It is an example of pharmacodynamics type of drug interaction.

Result of Interaction

- Possibility of precipitation of heart failure, atrioventricular (AV) block, and severe bradycardia.
- Compensation of bronchoconstrictory effect of propranolol by verapamil.

Mechanism of Interaction

- Both propranolol and verapamil reduce myocardial contractility, heart rate, and impulse conduction. In addition, verapamil inhibits hepatic metabolism of propranolol to some extent.
- Propranolol blocks $beta_2$ adrenergic receptors of the smooth muscle of trachal–bronchial tree and increases airway resistance. Verapamil by preventing calcium entry can cause bronchodilatation.

Remarks

Cotherapy should be done cautiously particularly in paroxysmal supraventricular tachycardia.

DIGOXIN AND HYDROCHLOROTHIAZIDE

Type

This is an example of pharmacodynamics type of drug interaction.

Result of Interaction

Precipitation of digoxin toxicity due to coadministration in the form of bradycardia and AV block.

Mechanism of Interaction

Digoxin is a cardiac glycoside used to treat heart failure with or without atrial fibrillation. Hydrochlorothiazide is a moderately potent diuretics used to treat hypertension and different cases of edema. Digoxin inhibits Na^+–K^+ ATPase pump of cardiac myocytes from outside. It binds to the outer phase of the enzyme, thereby inhibiting the efflux of sodium from within the cell. Accumulation of sodium will result in exchange with calcium and increase force of contraction. As long-term use of hydrochlorothiazide will produce hypokalemia, by inhibiting Na^+–K^+–$2Cl^-$ pump; so the binding of digoxin will be enhanced to its target. This may produce bradycardia and conduction blockade at AV node as features of cardiotoxicity.

Remarks

These two should not be coadministered.

CHLORPROPAMIDE AND DICOUMAROL

Type

It is a pharmacokinetic type of drug interaction at the level of drug metabolism.

Result of Interaction

Hypoglycemic effect of chlorpropamide is increased.

Mechanism of Interaction

Chlorpropamide is an oral hypoglycemic agent. Dicoumarol is an oral anticoagulant acting only *in vivo*. Dicoumarol prolongs the half-life of chlorpropamide by inhibiting its hepatic metabolism and/or reduced renal clearance of chlorpropamide.

Remarks

During cotherapy, the dose of chlorpropamide has to be adjusted.

GENTAMICIN AND GALLAMINE

Type

It is a pharmacodynamics type of drug interaction.

Result of Interaction

Muscle relaxant effect of gallamine is increased.

Mechanism of Interaction

Gentamicin is an aminoglycoside antibiotic while gallamine is a nondepolarizing neuromuscular blocking agent. Gallamine and acetyl choline compete for N_M receptors of motor end plate in the neuromuscular junction (NMJ) and relaxant effect of gallamine is reduced. Gentamicin inhibits acetylcholine (Ach) release from motor end plate and thus increases the relaxant effect of gallamine.

Remarks

- Gallamine should not be used with aminoglycoside antibiotics.
- If at all used together, the dose of gallamine should be reduced.

LITHIUM AND THIAZIDE

Type

It is an example of pharmacokinetic type of drug interaction.

Result of Interaction

Chance of lithium toxicity will be enhanced in a patient on long-standing thiazide therapy.

Mechanism of Interaction

Thiazides are sodium depleting diuretics which on long-term may lead to hyponatremia. This will be reflected in the form of low sodium content of proximal convoluted tubule fluid. If a patient has been taking along with thiazide, lithium ions; which share the same epithelial transporter as sodium ions will be reabsorbed in preference. This will lead to increased serum concentration of lithium and will precipitate symptoms of toxicity.

Remarks

These two drugs should not be coadministered. Amiloride is the ideal diuretic in this situation.

PROPRANOLOL AND INSULIN

Type

This is a pharmacodynamic type of drug interaction.

Results of Interaction

- Masking the effects of insulin induced hypoglycemia
- Potentiation of hypoglycemia
- Delayed recovery from hypoglycemia
- Increase in blood pressure and chance of angina precipitation.

Mechanism of Interaction

Propranolol is a nonselective beta-blocker used to treat various cardiological and noncardiological illnesses. Insulin is a hypoglycemic peptide hormone secreted from beta cells of pancreas.

- Hypoglycemia induced by insulin gives rise to compensatory sympathetic overactivity characterized by tachycardia, tremor, palpitation, sweating, and high blood pressure. As propranolol nonselectively blocks all the beta-receptors, so manifestations of these clinical features which occur via beta-receptor stimulation may be masked.

- Propranolol being a nonselective beta-blocker also blocks beta-3 metabotropic receptors leading to potentiation of insulin-induced hypoglycemia.
- Compensatory sympathetic overactivity induced by hypoglycemia initiates hepatic glycogenolysis in a normal person. However in presence of propranolol, it will remain blocked.
- Unopposed action of catecholamines on alpha-receptors may give rise to high blood pressure and precipitate angina.

Remarks

Propranolol should be replaced by cardioselective beta-blockers in patients receiving insulin.

ENALAPRIL AND SPIRONOLACTONE

Type

This is an example of pharmacodynamic type of drug interaction.

Result of Interaction

Dangerous level of hyperkalemia may be precipitated resulting in cardiac arrhythmias.

Mechanism of Interaction

Enalapril is an ACEi prodrug used to treat hypertension and congestive cardiac failure. Spironolactone is a moderately potent potassium sparing diuretic. Enalapril blocks the conversion of angiotensin I to angiotensin II that ultimately stimulates aldosterone secretion from suprarenal cortex. Aldosterone acts on late distal convoluted tubule and collecting ducts by entering epithelial cells from basolateral side, combines with cytosolic receptors and is translocated to nuclear DNA. This stimulates the production of aldosterone induced protein which then increases luminal sodium ion transporter as well basolateral potassium channel. Increased amount of sodium influx from tubular lumen into the epithelial cells will be balanced by efflux of potassium and hydrogen ions from within the cell. Spironolactone selectively blocks cytosolic aldosterone receptor and the whole process is blocked resulting in preservation of potassium ions and precipitation of dangerous hyperkalemia.

Remarks

These two drugs should not be coadministered.

CHAPTER

12

Pharmacology Charts

Avishek Layek, Dyuti Deepta Rano

Note:
This table in final examination contains 3–5 marks.
Firstly, the student needs to identify the chart and describe it. That is followed by some related questions.

CHARTS

Three types of charts are described here.

Log Dose-response Curves

The dose-response curve is a simple X-Y graph relating the magnitude of a stressor to the response of a receptor. The response may be physiological or biochemical or even death (as in mortality studies). The measured dose is plotted on the *X*-axis and the response on the *Y*-axis. There are two types of responses: (i) graded, and (ii) all-or-none.

For example, in a study for blood pressure (BP) reduction with a new drug, there may be a study measuring reduction in BP in absolute terms. Another study may place a cut off (say 10% pretreatment reduction) and just determine whether candidates are responders or nonresponders.

Plotting graded response produces sigmoid shaped curves whereas all-or-none responses produce quantal or bell shaped curves (Figs 12.1 and 12.2).

Figure 12.3 is a chart showing graded log dose-response curves of an agonist in presence and absence of a competitive antagonist.

1. Why competitive?

Because with increasing concentration of antagonist, the curve retains its maximal height and only shifts parallel to the right.

- Examples of competitive antagonists—
  - Acetylcholine and atropine on muscarinic receptors.
  - Acetylcholine and D-tubocurarine on N_m receptors.
  - Acetylcholine and hexamethonium on N_n receptors.

Figure 12.4 is a chart showing graded log dose-response curves of an agonist in presence and absence of a noncompetitive antagonist.

2. Why noncompetitive?

The tracing shows that the log dose–response curves of the agonist become nonparallel and there is diminution of maximal response.

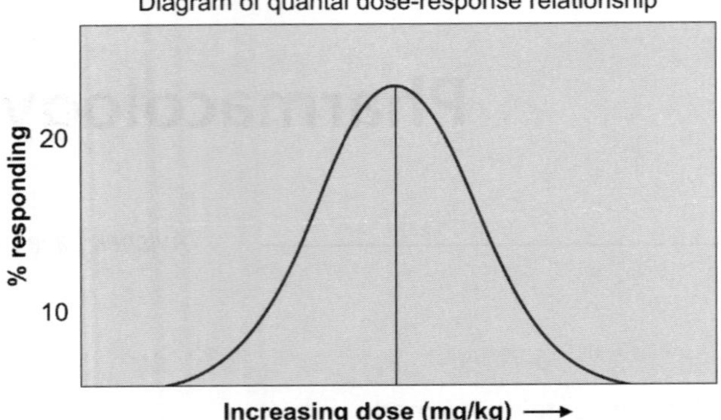

Fig. 12.1: Quantal curve example (only option for contraceptives)

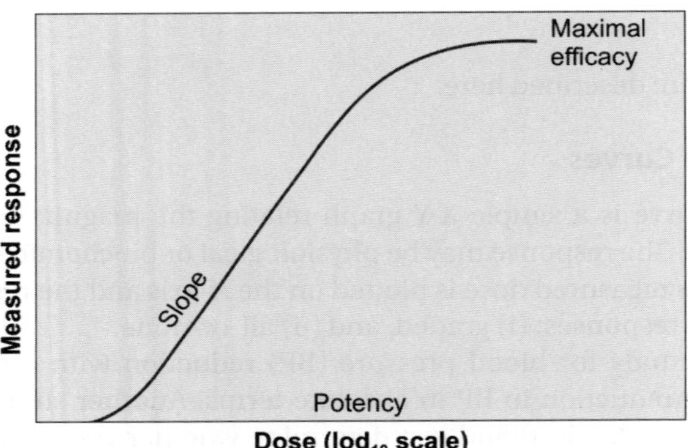

Fig. 12.2: Sigmoid curve

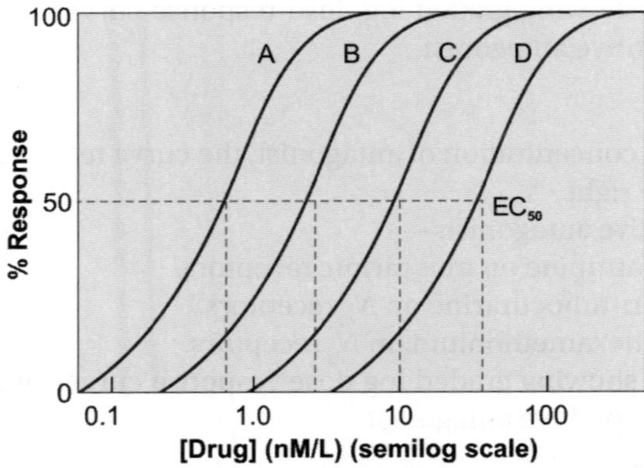

Fig. 12.3: Graded log-dose response curves of an agonist in presence and absence of a competitive antagonist. Curve A shows response in absence of antagonist. Curves B to D show response in presence of increasing concentrations of antagonist

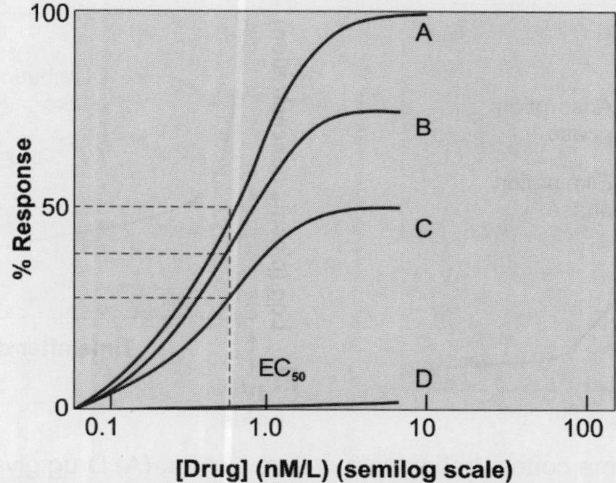

Fig. 12.4: Graded log-dose response curves of an agonist in presence and absence of a noncompetitive antagonist. Curve A shows response in absence of antagonist. Curves B to D show response in presence of increasing concentrations of antagonist

- Examples of noncompetitive:
  - Acetylcholine and alpha-bungarotoxin on N_m receptors.
  - Adrenaline/noradrenaline and phenoxybenzamine on alpha adrenergic receptors.

Plasma Concentration versus Time Curves (Figs. 12.5A and B)

Shapes of these curves depend upon the route of administration of the drug. Plasma concentration is plotted in *Y*-axis and time in *X*-axis.

They have the following uses:

- These curves offer an idea about the pharmacokinetic pattern of the drugs and that knowledge can be utilized in therapy.
- To calculate C_{max} (defined as maximum concentration achieved in plasma).
- To calculate T_{max} (time required to reach C_{max}).
- To calculate volume of distribution.
- To calculate plasma $T_{1/2}$ (half-life).
- To calculate bioavailability.

Types of pharmacokinetic models are compartment models, noncompartment models and physiological models.

Compartment models: These are classical pharmacological models that simulate the kinetic processes of drug absorption, distribution, and elimination against time with little physiologic detail. It is of two types:

- *Open models*: The drug is eliminated by some excretory mechanism.
- *Closed models*: The drug is not eliminated.

Figure 12.5A is a chart showing a plasma concentration versus time curve of a drug given by oral route with the drug showing gradual increase in concentration after administration and then after reaching the peak, there is a gradual decline.

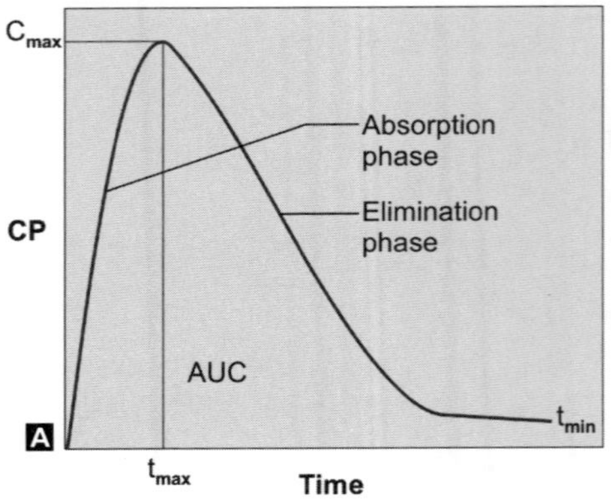

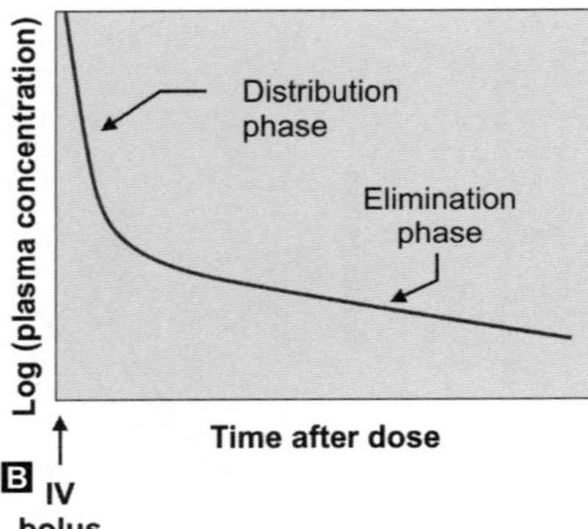

Figs. 12.5A and B: Plasma concentration versus time curves. (A) Drug given by oral route with the drug showing gradual increase in concentration after administration and then after reaching the peak, there is a gradual decline. (B) Drug given by intravenous route with the drug showing nonuniform decline in plasma concentration with time

3. Why oral?

Peak concentration is preceded by a phase of gradual increase suggesting absorption.

4. Is there any other possibility?

- This type of curve may also be obtained following any depot injection, such as in intramuscular (IM) or subcutaneous (SC) route.

Figure 12.5B is a chart showing a plasma concentration versus time curve of a drug given by intravenous (IV) route with the drug showing nonuniform decline in plasma concentration with time, suggesting that the drug follows two-compartment model.

5. Why intravenous?

Because the maximum concentration is achieved at 0 hours.

- Example of drugs showing two-compartment model—
  - Thiopentone sodium and diazepam IV.

6. What is two-compartment model?

This is an open type of model, where the body is assumed to be having two-compartments: a central and a peripheral. The central compartment represents highly perfused tissues [blood and extracellular fluid (ECF)], whereas the peripheral represents the poorly perfused tissues (fatty tissues).

The decline is thus biexponential and is the sum of two first order processes, i.e. distribution and elimination.

The plasma concentration declines in two phases:

1. *Initial rapid or alpha phase:* In this phase, distribution of the drug from central compartment to periphery predominates.
2. *Slow or beta phase:* In this phase, elimination of the drug predominates.

Figure 12.6 is a chart showing a plasma concentration versus time curve of a drug given by intravenous route with the drug showing uniform decline in plasma concentration with time, suggesting that the drug follows one-compartment model.

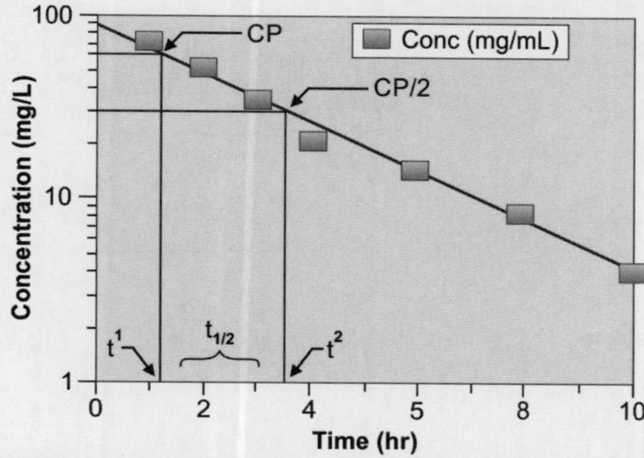

Fig. 12.6: Plasma concentration versus time curve of a drug given by intravenous route with the drug showing uniform decline suggesting that the drug follows one-compartment model

7. Why intravenous?

Because the maximum concentration is achieved at 0 hours.

8. What is one-compartment model?

This is an open type of model, where the body is assumed to be a single kinetically homogeneous unit with no barriers to movement of the drug. Drug elimination in this model always follows first order kinetics.

9. Classify one compartment model?

- IV bolus
- IV infusion
- Extravascular first order absorption.

Kymographic Tracings

A kymograph (a Greek-derived word meaning *wave writer*) is a device that draws a graphical representation of spatial position over time. Basically, it consists of a revolving drum wrapped with a sheet of paper on which a *stylus* moves back and forth, thus recording perceived changes of the phenomenon under observation (Fig. 12.7).

Kymographic tracings are obtained on a sheet of paper wrapped around the drum and are of two types:

1. *Positive tracing:* Here the paper is blank and the stylus is inked (Fig. 12.8).
2. *Negative tracing:* Here the paper is smoked and the stylus has no ink; rather it only produces etchings on the smoked paper (Fig. 12.9).

Out of the two, negative tracings are more accurate as positive tracings provide more resistance during fine movements of stylus.

Figures 12.10A and B show the copies of positive/negative (as given) kymographic tracing of mean arterial blood pressure of anesthetized cat following administration of a pressor agent like noradrenaline or angiotensin and adrenaline, respectively. There is initial rise is blood pressure followed by normalization.

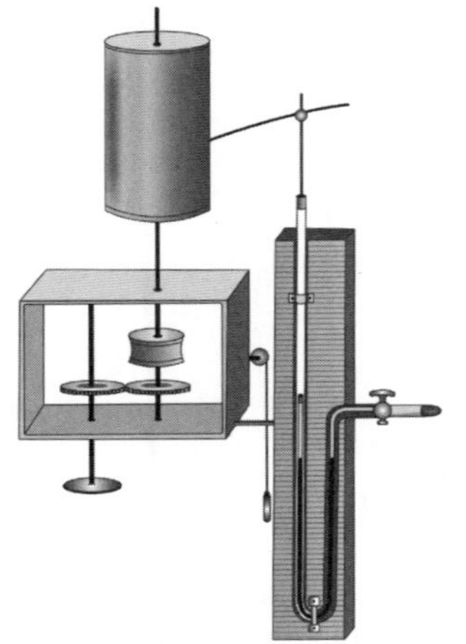

Fig. 12.7: A kymograph recording changes in pressure via a manometer

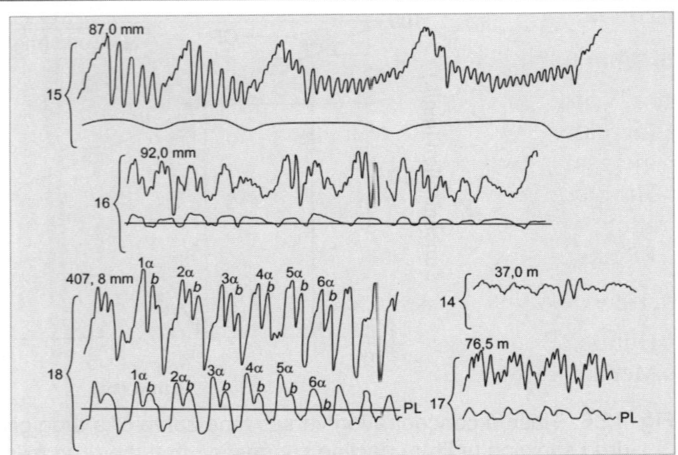

Fig. 12.8: Positive tracing

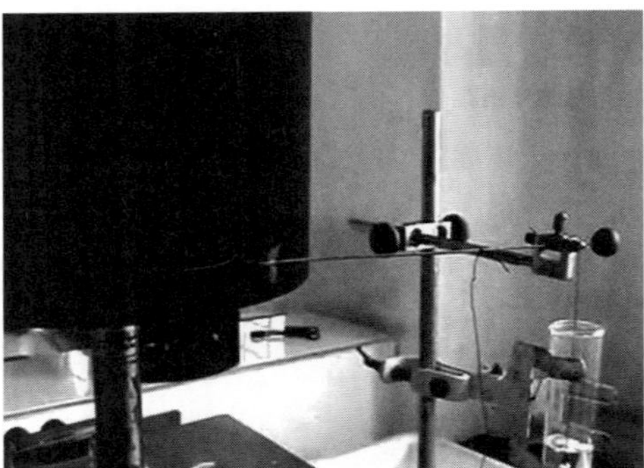

Fig. 12.9: Negative tracing

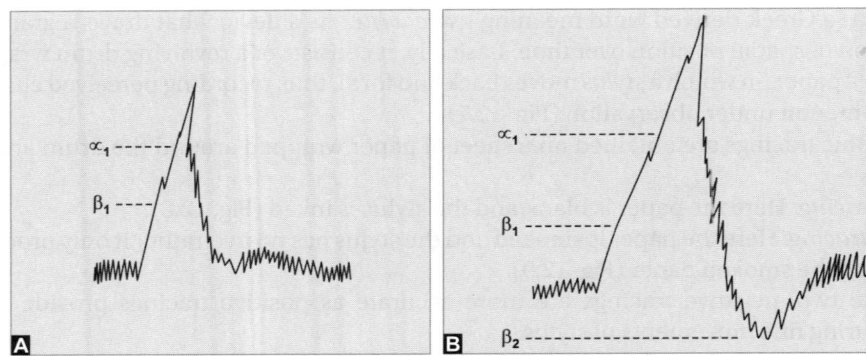

Figs. 12.10A and B: Graphs show the positive/negative (as given) kymographic tracing of mean arterial blood pressure of anesthetized cat following administration of a pressor agent like—(A) noradrenaline or angiotensin; (B) adrenaline. There is initial rise is blood pressure followed by normalization

Discussion

10. What is the Reason of rise in BP?

After IV administration, following mechanisms increase the BP:

- Increases the force of contraction of heart as well as heart rate by beta-1 receptors, thus increasing cardiac output.
- The blood vessels of the skin and mucous membranes are constricted due to alpha receptor stimulation, thereby increasing peripheral vascular resistance (PVR).
- BP rises, as it is the product of cardiac output and PVR.

11. How does normalization take place?

- Dilution by diffusion
- Metabolism by L-monoamine oxidases (MAO) and catechol-O-methyltransferase (COMT) enzymes.

12. How to differentiate between adrenaline and noradrenaline?

- *By heart rate*, reflex bradycardia suggests noradrenaline while tachycardia suggests adrenaline
- *By administration of alpha-blocker*, adrenaline but not noradrenaline will show vasomotor reversal of dale.
- *During normalization*, the curve in case of adrenaline goes below baseline due to beta-2 vasodilatory action leading to lowering of PVR.

Figure 12.11 is a copy of positive/negative (as given) kymographic tracing of mean arterial blood pressure of anesthetized cat following administration of different drugs.

Discussion

13. Why there is resetting of mean arterial BP at a lower level?

Alpha-blockers lead to persistent fall of BP.

14. Why there is fall instead of rise with adrenaline when given after alpha-blocker?

Adrenaline has beta-2 vasodilatory action leading to lowering of PVR. With the alpha-constrictory action abolished by alpha-blocker, beta-2 action overpowers and causes fall in BP.

15. How to define vasomotor reversal of Dale?

This is the phenomenon of reversal of pressor response of adrenaline to depressor one after prior administration of alpha adrenergic blocking agent.

16. What is the response of phenylephrine after alpha-blocker?

The pressor action is completely abolished but there is no fall in BP.

17. Does noradrenaline show vasomotor reversal of Dale?

It has no beta-2 adrenergic vasodilatory activity. Moreover, there is residual beta-1 pressor action.

18. What is reversal of vasomotor reversal of Dale?

If after vasomotor reversal of Dale has been demonstrated, a nonselective beta-blocker like propranolol is administered; then repetition of adrenaline causes neither fall nor rise in BP. This is called reversal of vasomotor reversal of Dale.

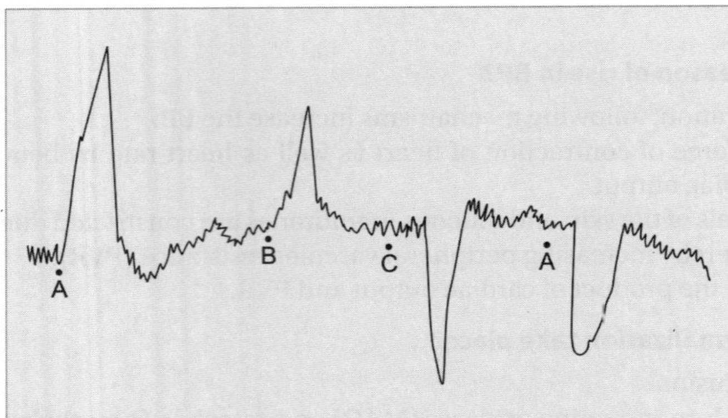

Fig. 12.11: Graph shows the positive/negative (as given) kymographic tracing of mean arterial blood pressure of anesthetized cat following administration of different drugs. The graph shows normal tracing before 1st dot (A). IV drug is given at 1st dot (A), after which there is sharp rise in BP. The normalization includes a fall below baseline suggesting adrenaline. Another IV drug was given at 2nd point (B), after which there is sharp rise in BP. The normalization does not include a fall below baseline suggesting noradrenaline. Another IV drug was given at 3rd point (C), after which there is sharp fall and quick normalization in BP, suggestive of acetylcholine/histamine/isoprenaline. Another IV drug was given at 4th point (D). At 5th point, drug A was repeated and this time there was fall in BP instead of rise. This is suggestive of drug D being alpha adrenergic blocker like dihydroergotoxine, phenoxybenzamine or phentolamine. This phenomenon is called vasomotor reversal of Dale

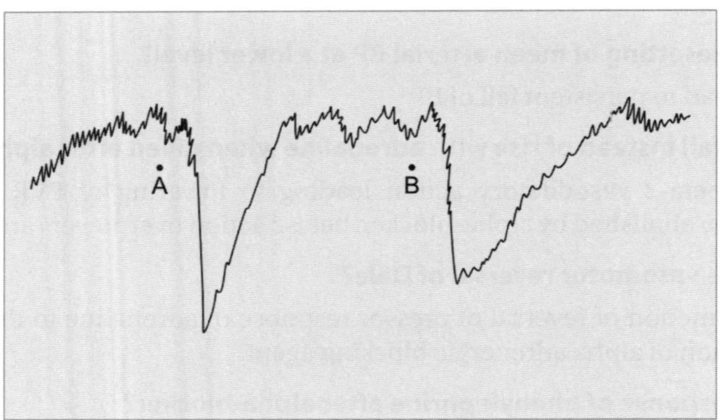

Fig. 12.12: Graph shows the positive/negative (as given) kymographic tracing of mean arterial blood pressure of anesthetized cat showing Initial normal BP tracing. At point A, one drug was given IV which caused sharp fall of BP and quick normalization suggesting acetylcholine/histamine. At point B, another drug was given IV which caused sharp fall of BP and gradual normalization suggesting methacholine/carbachol/physostigmine/bethanechol

Figure 12.12 shows the copy of positive/negative (as given) kymographic tracing of mean arterial blood pressure of anesthetized cat.

Discussion

19. Why delayed normalization after drug at point (B)?

Carbachol and bethanechol are not metabolized by cholinesterases. Methacholine is slowly metabolized by true cholinesterase but is resistant to pseudocholinesterase. Physostigmine inhibits acetylcholinesterase, so that residence time of acetylcholine at neuromuscular junction (NMJ) is increased.

20. If all drugs are cholinergic, fall of BP indicates what type of response?

Muscarinic response:

Figure 12.13 shows the copy of positive/negative (as given) kymographic tracing of mean arterial blood pressure of anesthetized cat.

Conclusion

- The first drug is acetylcholine (1–5 µg per kg body weight)
- The second drug is atropine (1 mg per kg body weight)
- The first drug is repeated in a dose of 0.5 mg/kg body weight
- The first depressor response is the muscarinic response whereas the later pressor response is called ganglionic nicotinic response.

Explanation

Initially fall in BP is due to vasodilatation mediated by vascular muscarinic M_3 receptors. Atropine blocks all muscarinic receptors but itself produces insignificant fall due to paradoxical vasodilatation. The repetition of high dose (50–100 times initial dose) of acetylcholine leads to stimulation of the autonomic ganglionic nicotinic receptors (N_N) at the following sites:

- N_N receptors at parasympathetic ganglion, which results in release of acetylcholine from the postganglionic nerve terminal. However, expected fall in BP is prevented by muscarinic block due to previously given atropine.

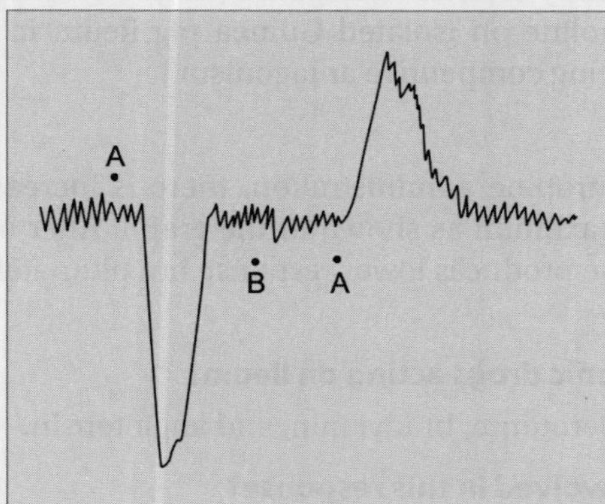

Fig. 12.13: Graph shows the positive/negative (as given) kymographic tracing of mean arterial blood pressure of anesthetized cat showing initial normal BP tracing At point A, a drug was administered and there is a sharp fall of BP and quick normalization. At point B, another drug was administered and caused insignificant alteration of BP. At the 3rd point, 1st drug was repeated at high dose and there was sharp rise and gradual normalization of BP

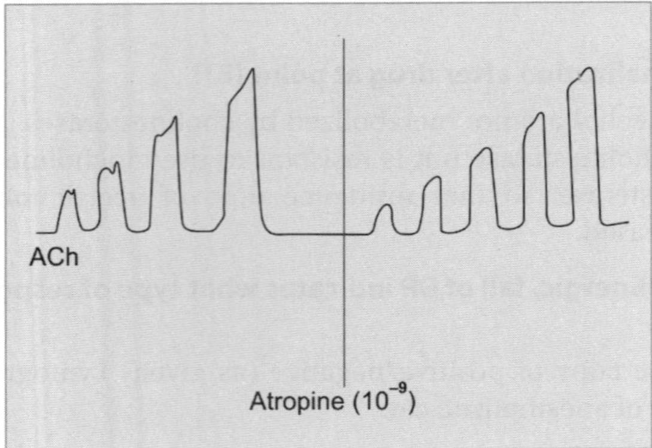

Fig. 12.14: Graph shows the positive/negative (as given) kymographic tracing of graded dose-response of acetyl choline on isolated guinea pig ileum in absence and presence of antagonist: Atropine showing competitive antagonism

- N_N receptors at sympathetic ganglion, which results in noradrenaline from postganglionic nerve terminal. It acts on alpha-adrenergic receptors causing vasoconstriction resulting in increased PVR and increased BP.
- N_N receptors at chromaffin cells of adrenal medulla, causing the gradual release of adrenaline and there is rising phase of BP followed by a gradual reduction.

Discussion

21. How nicotinic response may be abolished?

By administration of ganglionic blocking agents like hexamethonium.

22. Why high dose of acetylcholine is needed?

Low dose of acetylcholine is not accessible to the autonomic ganglion.

Figure 12.14 shows the copy of positive/negative (as given) kymographic tracing of Graded dose response of acetylcholine on isolated Guinea pig ileum in absence and presence of antagonist—atropine showing competitive antagonism.

23. Why competitive?

Left of the line showing atropine administration, there is increase in contractile response to acetylcholine up to a maximum as shown in the graph. After administration of atropine, same doses of acetylcholine produces lower response but ultimately the maximal response is attained.

24. Name some spasmogenic drugs acting on ileum?

Acetylcholine, histamine, serotonin, bradykinin, and angiotensin.

25. Which receptors are involved in this response?

Muscarinic M_3 receptors are involved in this response.

26. How will this curve look if plotted graphically?

Such as Figure 12.2. (Sigmoid dose-response curve with right parallel shifting only and without any alteration in slope or maximal height).

CHAPTER 13

Spotting in Pharmacology

Avishek Layek

1. Blister/ordinary ALU strip containing coated/uncoated scored/unscored ______ colored timed/sustained/controlled release tablet.

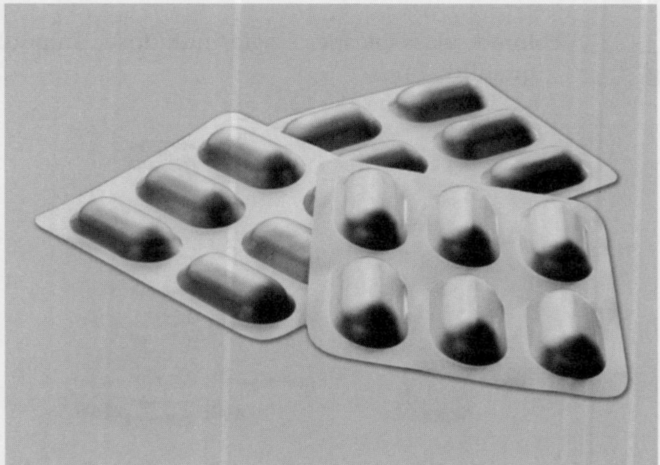

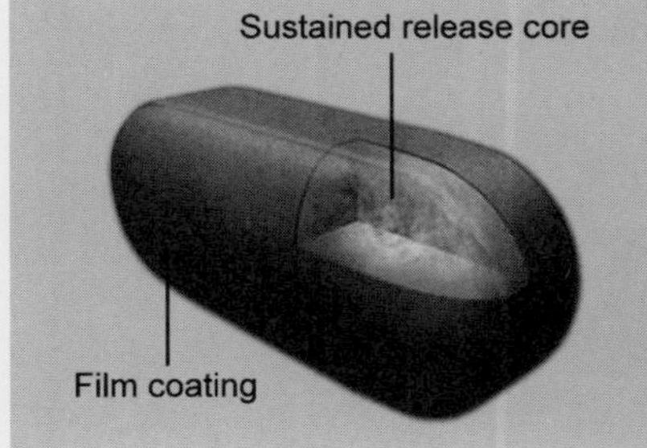

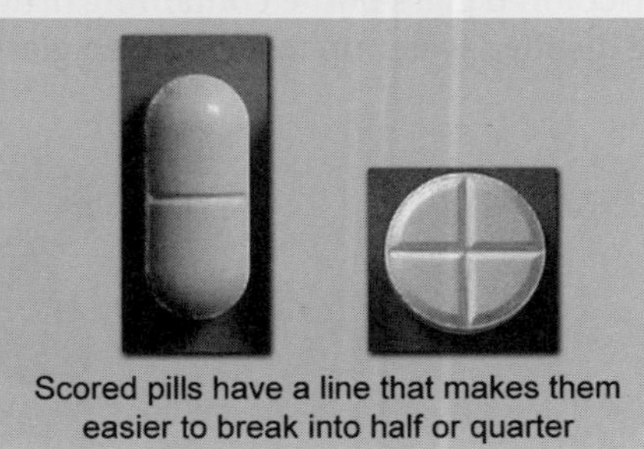

2. Blister/ordinary ALU strip containing hard/soft gelatin Transparent/_______colored timed/sustained/controlled release capsules.

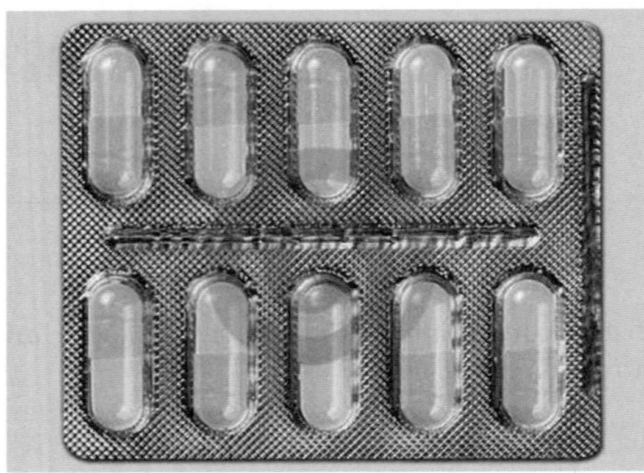

3. Transparent/_______ colored glass/plastic single/multidose ampoule/vial-containing injectable drug ________ quantity__ mL.

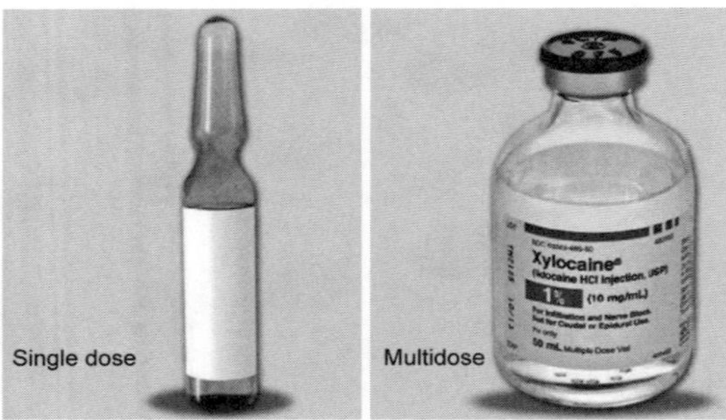

4. Amber-colored glass bottle containing drug_____ in the powder form for reconstitution by adding distilled water up to a specified glass marking.

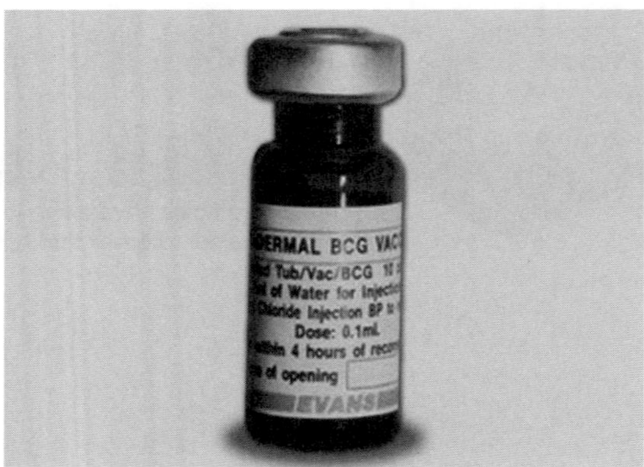

5. Metered dose inhaler (with/without cap)

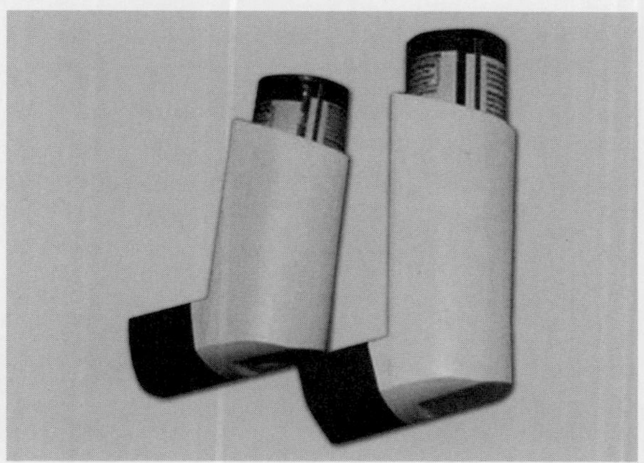

6. Lupihaler

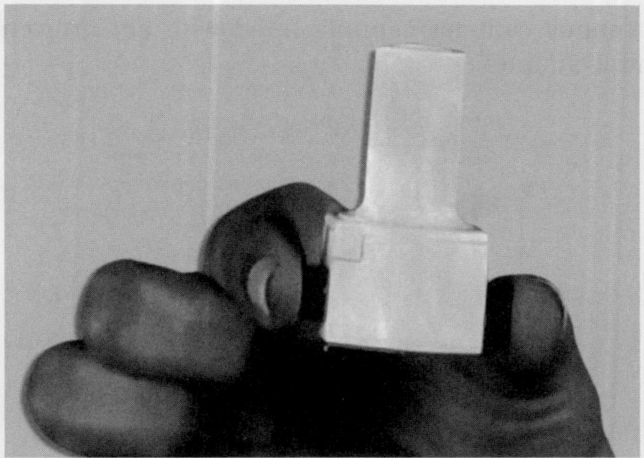

7. ___mL plastic/glass-prefilled syringe fitted with an intravenous/intradermal needle of ________ (name of drug). (May not be fitted with needle)

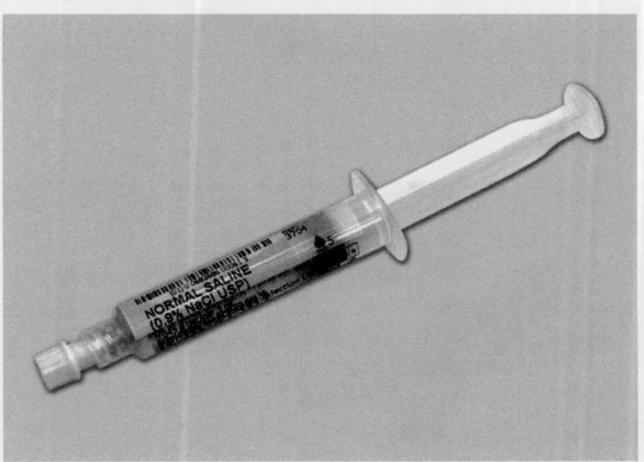

8. Malleable intravenous catheter/cannula fitted with an intravenous stellate.

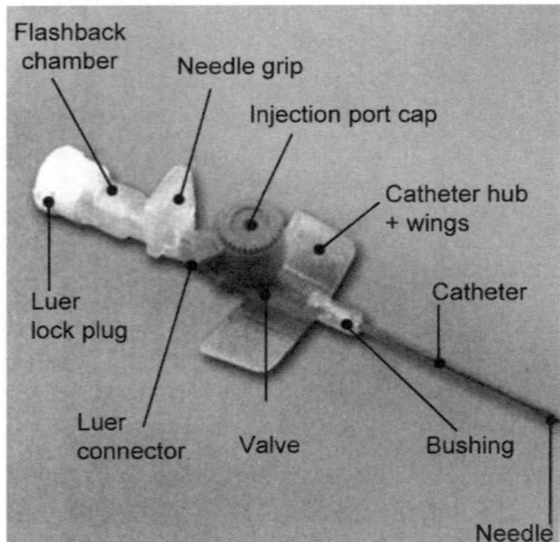

9. Malleable intravenous catheter/cannula fitted with an intravenous stellate used for preparing a central channel.

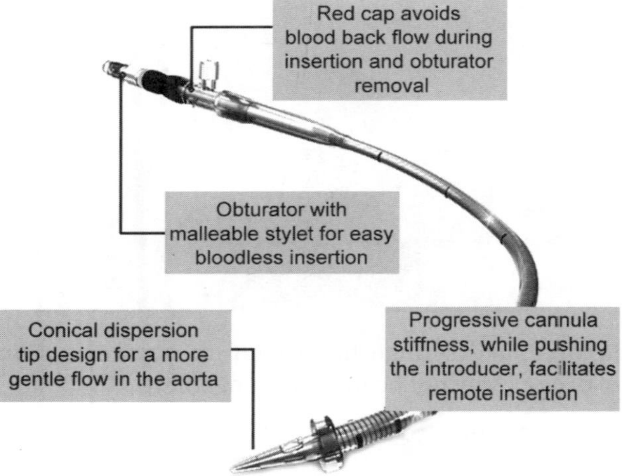

10. Metallic collapsible ointment tube containing______.

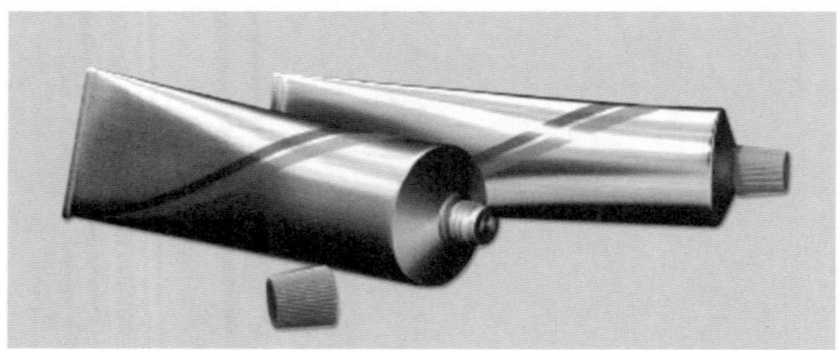

11. Disposable sterile blood transfusion set (check filter inside drip chamber)

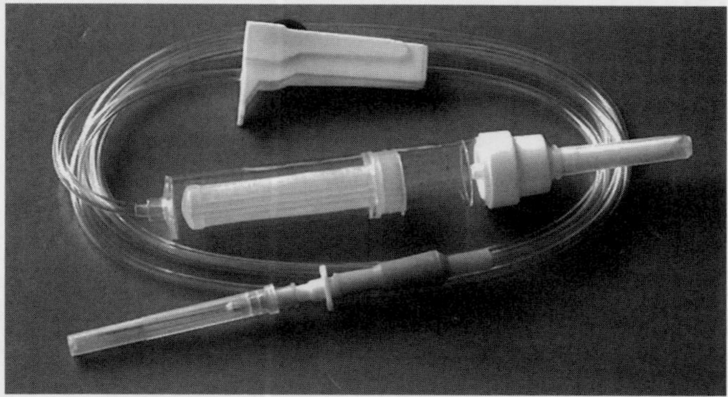

12. Disposable sterile intravenous fluid infusion set.

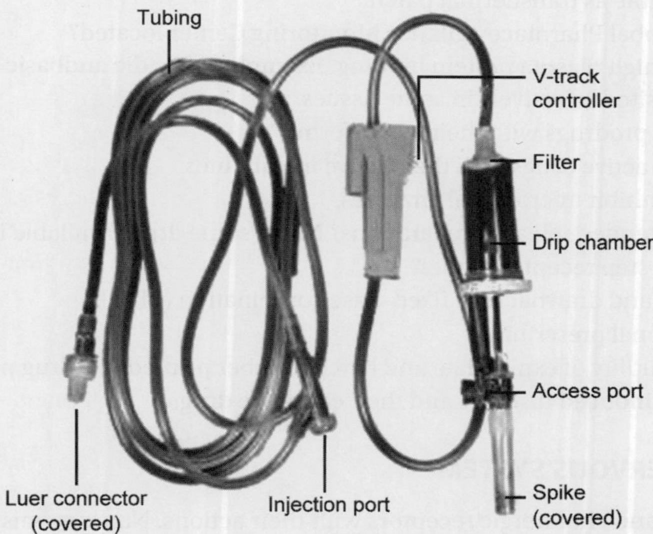

Component of an IV fluid therapy set

CHAPTER 14

Important Viva Questions

Avishek Layek, Dyuti Deepta Rano

GENERAL PHARMACOLOGY

1. All definitions from Chapter 1.
2. What are sources of drug information?
3. Drugs available as transdermal patch.
4. Where is Global Pharmacovigilance Monitoring Center located?
5. Drugs with high plasma protein binding. Examples of acidic andbasic binding.
6. Drugs deposited selectively in some tissues.
7. Name some prodrugs with their active forms.
8. Name some active drugs with their active metabolites.
9. Drugs that inhibit microsomal enzymes.
10. What are extended release preparations? Name some drugs available in that form.
11. What is two-step receptor model?
12. Advantages and drawbacks of fixed-dose combination (FDC).
13. What is rational prescribing?
14. What is the utility of expiry date and batch number printed in a drug packet?
15. Name drug-induced diseases and their causative drugs.

AUTONOMIC NERVOUS SYSTEM

16. Adrenergic and cholinergic receptors with their actions. Name agonist and antagonists of each type.
17. What is cotransmission?
18. Drugs affecting cholinergic transmission.
19. Uses of botulinum toxin.
20. Treatment of myasthenia gravis.
21. What is edrophonium challenge test?
22. Name ganglionic blocking agents.
23. Drugs affecting adrenergic transmission.
24. Name some anorectic agents.
25. Uses of beta-blockers including central uses.
26. Antiobesity drugs (Chapter 15)
27. Basic pathology in two types of glaucoma and their line of management.

AUTACOIDS

28. Define autacoid.
29. Effects of histamine.
30. Histaminic receptors, their agonist and antagonists.
31. Advantages of second-generation antihistaminics over first-generation.
32. Why are antihistaminics ineffective in bronchial asthma?
33. Name some drugs used for vertigo.
34. Drugs affecting serotonergic transmission.
35. Drugs used for migraine prophylaxis.
36. What is status migrainosus? Treatment?
37. Uses of prostaglandin (PG) analogs?
38. Uses of platelet-activating factor (PAF) antagonists?
39. What is Reye's syndrome?
40. Analgesic, antipyretic and anti-inflammatory doses of aspirin with indications?
41. Side effects and drug interactions of nonsteroidal anti-inflammatory drugs (NSAIDs).
42. Problems with COX2 inhibitors.
43. Name some topical NSAIDs.
44. What are disease-modifying antirheumatic drugs (DMARDS)?
45. Name some IL-1 antagonists.
46. Name drugs used in gout.
47. Drug of choice for hyperuricemia of tumor lysis syndrome (Rasburicase).

RESPIRATORY

48. Name some cough suppressants.
49. Name some long-acting beta-2 agonists.
50. Name anti-IgE antibody used in asthma.
51. What are status asthmaticus and its treatment?
52. What are spacer and nebulizer?

HORMONES

53. Uses of octreotide and bromocriptine.
54. How is thyroid hormone synthesized? What are active forms?
55. What are the uses of thyroid hormone (fT4)?
56. Difference between propylthiouracil and carbimazole.
57. What are goitrogens?
58. Uses of radioactive iodine (diagnostic and therapeutic).
59. What is thyroid storm, thyroid escape, thyroid constipation, Wolff–Chaikoff effect?
60. Chemical structure and synthesis of insulin.
61. What is first pass effect of insulin? How can oral insulin be helpful?
62. Why can insulin glargine not be mixed with any other preparation?
63. What preparation is used in CSII?
64. What is split mixed regime and basal-bolus regime?
65. Name some new insulin delivery routes and devices.
66. Other use of metformin than diabetes.

67. Uses of glucagon.
68. Name some hyperglycemics.
69. What are the glucocorticoid and mineralocorticoid actions of steroids?
70. Which steroids are used in cerebral edema?
71. Uses of fludrocortisone.
72. Name a male contraceptive drug.
73. What is hormone replacement therapy (HRT)?
74. Uses of selective estrogen receptor modulator (SERM), selective progesterone receptor modulator (SPRM), and aromatase inhibitors.
75. Uses of ormeloxifene.
76. Name some tocolytics.
77. Uses of vitamin D and bisphosphonates.

PERIPHERAL NERVOUS SYSTEM

78. What is depolarizing and nondepolarizing block? Name drugs.
79. What is phase I and II block?
80. Why is atracurium used even in hepatic and renal insufficiency?
81. Use of dantrolene sodium.
82. Difference between central and peripheral acting muscle relaxants.
83. Uses of lignocaine.
84. What is eutectic mixture of local anesthetics (EMLA)?
85. What is IV regional anesthesia and spinal anesthesia?
86. Why is adrenaline mixed with lignocaine?
87. Shortest-acting competitive blocker: Mivacurium.

CENTRAL NERVOUS SYSTEM

88. What are minimum alveolar concentration (MAC), diffusion hypoxia, and second gas effect?
89. Properties of ideal anesthetic.
90. What is malignant hyperthermia?
91. Effect of IV anesthetics on vital functions.
92. Preanesthetic medications.
93. What is conscious sedation?
94. Use of fomepizole.
95. What is disulfiram reaction?
96. Difference between sedative and hypnotic.
97. Benzodiazepines (BZD) versus barbiturates.
98. Drugs affecting $GABA_A$ receptor.
99. Use of flumazenil and ramelteon.
100. Define epilepsy and status epilepticus.
101. Side effects of phenytoin.
102. Uses of valproate.
103. Uses of levodopa.
104. What is ON/OFF phenomenon and drug holiday?
105. Advantages of second-generation antipsychotics.

106. Uses of lithium.
107. Possible benefits of cannabinoids.
108. Uses of opioid analogs.
109. Treatment of morphine withdrawal.
110. Same some endogenous opioid peptides and their physiological significance.
111. Uses of rivastigmine.
112. Name some cognitive enhancers.

CARDIOVASCULAR

113. What is renin–angiotensin system (RAS)?
114. Significance of hexapeptide angiotensin IV (Ang IV)?
115. Classify inhibitors of RAS.
116. Kinin receptors and their significance.
117. Digoxin—use, mechanism of action (MOA), side effect, antibody
118. Congestive heart failure (CHF) and acute myocardial infarction (AMI) treatment.
119. PDE 3 inhibitors.
120. Drugs causing torsades de pointes.
121. Drug of choice of AF, AFL and PSVT.
122. Types of angina and its pathophysiology.
123. Nitrates—uses, MOA, drug interactions, tolerance, cross tolerance, dependence.
124. Calcium-channel blockers—types of calcium channel, uses, side effects (cause of edema).
125. Clonidine—learn everything.
126. Antihypertensive choices according to age.
127. Ultra short-acting beta blocker: Esmolol.

RENAL

128. Free water clearance.
129. Why high ceiling diuretics are named so? Name some of them. What are their uses?
130. Paradoxical effect of thiazide in type 1 DM?
131. Use of metolazone.
132. Uses of acetazolamide and mannitol.
133. Mechanism of action of vasopressin.
134. Uses of desmopressin.
135. Name some vasopressin antagonists and their uses.
136. Drugs used for type 1 DM (Chapter 15).
137. What are potassium-sparing diuretics? What is their significance and uses?

BLOOD AND BLOOD FORMATION

138. Define hematinics. Name some conventional and unconventional hematinics.
139. What are the available iron preparations for oral and parenteral therapy?
140. Daily requirements of iron.
141. What is ferritin curtain?
142. Indications and side effects of parenteral iron therapy?

143. Acute iron poisoning treatment
144. Uses of vitamin B_{12} and folic acid
145. Use erythropoietin (EPO).
146. Name some coagulants and anticoagulants.
147. Contraindications of heparin.
148. Advantages and uses of low-molecular-weight heparin (LMWH).
149. *Oral direct thrombin inhibitor*: Dabigatran etexilate.
150. Uses of fibrinolytics.
151. Name some antifibrinolytics.
152. Classify antiplatelet drugs and enumerate uses.
153. Classify hypolipidemics.
154. Why are some statins given at night only and some at any time of day?
155. Name some plasma expanders and their uses.
156. Desirable properties of a plasma expander.
157. Name some fibrates and their uses.

GASTROINTESTINAL

158. What are the neurotransmitters of enteric nervous system?
159. How is gastric acid secretion regulated?
160. Why is ranitidine still preferred over PPIs in some situations?
161. Uses of PPIs and H_2 blockers.
162. Name some antacids and their combinations.
163. MOA and use of sucralfate and colloidal bismuth subcitrate (CBS).
164. Anti-*H. pylori* regimen.
165. Drugs used for GERD.
166. Name some emetics and antiemetics.
167. Name some digestants and gallstone dissolving drugs.
168. Laxative vs Purgative. Examples and uses.
169. Lactulose in hepatic encephalopathy
170. Nonspecific antidiarrheal drugs and probiotics in diarrhea.
171. Antimotility drugs—names and uses.
172. Uses of sulfasalazine.

ANTIMICROBIALS

173. Define AMA, antibiotic, superinfection, MIC, MBC, PAE and supra-additive effect.
174. Disadvantages of antimicrobial combinations.
175. Causes of failure of AMA therapy.
176. Cotrimoxazole.
177. Drugs for typhoid fever.
178. Fluoroquinolones: Uses, names, bioavailability.
179. Classify penicillins and what are their MOA and side effects.
180. Antipseudomonal penicillin, anti-MRSA, anti-VRSA drugs.
181. Fifth generation cephalosporins: Ceftobiprole, ceftaroline, and ceftolozane.
182. What are monobactams and carbapenems?
183. MOA of aminoglycosides, tetracyclines, chloramphenicol and erythromycin.

184. Side effects and uses of tetracycline and chloramphenicol.
185. Common properties of aminoglycosides and their uses.
186. *Macrolides*: Uses, names, side effects.
187. *Linezolid*: Uses, spectrum.
188. Name some urinary antiseptics.
189. *Antitubercular and antimalarial drugs*: Read virtually everything.
190. *Dapsone and Clofaziminbe*: MOA, dosage, adverse effects.
191. Multidrug therapy (MDT) of leprosy.
192. *Amp-B and ketoconazole*: MOA, uses and side effects.
193. Topical antifungals.
194. Highly active antiretroviral therapy (HAART)
195. *Acyclovir*: MOA, uses.
196. Ritonavir boosted therapy.
197. Human immunodeficiency virus (HIV) prophylaxis
198. *Nitroimidazoles*: Names, MOA, uses.
199. Mebendazole, albendazole—uses and dose.
200. Praziquantel and DEC—uses, MOA.
201. What is apparent antagonism?
202. Name some antimicrobial anticancer drugs.

CHEMOTHERAPY

203. Cisplatin, methotrexate, azathioprine: MOA, uses and side effects.
204. Cell cycle specific agents.
205. General principles of chemotherapy in cancer.
206. Use of filgrastim.
207. Uses of thalidomide.

MISCELLANEOUS

208. Name some immunosuppressants and immune-modulants.
209. Anti-acne drugs.
210. What is occlusive dressing and its use?
211. *Penicillamine, desferrioxamine*: MOA and uses.
212. *Oral iron chelator*: Deferiprone, deferasirox.
213. Vaccine versus sera versus toxoid.

CHAPTER

15

Miscellaneous Notes

Avishek Layek, Dyuti Deepta Rano

1. Diagnostic Uses of Drugs

- **Radiopaque dyes**: Barium, urografin, etc.
- Oral glucose tolerance test.
- Desmopressin challenge test.
- Dexamethasone challenge test.
- **Clomiphene challenge test**: To test for fertility.
- **Bronchial challenge test**: Using nebulised methacholine or histamine.
- **Ameliorative test for myasthenia gravis**: Edrophonium.
- **Provocative test for myasthenia gravis**: d-tubocurarine.
- **Salbutamol**: To distinguish between obstructive and restrictive pulmonary disease.
- **Ajmaline test**: To diagnose arrhythmia (Brugada syndrome) by provocating ECG changes.
- **DEC provocation test**: To diagnose filariasis.
- **Provocative test for glaucoma**: Using short acting mydriatic like phenylephrine.
- **Water drinking test for glaucoma**: Tonometry before and after to confirm glaucoma.
- Antibiotics for sensitivity testing, e.g. penicillin.
- Sensitivity testing in microbiological cultures.

2. Indications of Therapeutic Drug Monitoring

- Sample to be taken just before next dose after steady state has been achieved:
  - Drugs with low safety margin, e.g. digoxin, lithium, TCAs, etc.
  - If individual pharmacokinetic variations are large, e.g. vancomycin, anti-depressants, etc.
  - Potentially toxic drugs used in presence of renal/hepatic failure.
  - In case of failure of therapy without any apparent reason.
- In case of drug poisoning: Sample taken as early as possible.
- To check patient compliance in doubtful cases: Random sampling.

3. Antibacterial Drugs Acting on Cell Membrane

The following figure shows the biosynthesis of cell wall peptidoglacan showing the sites of action of five antibiotics.

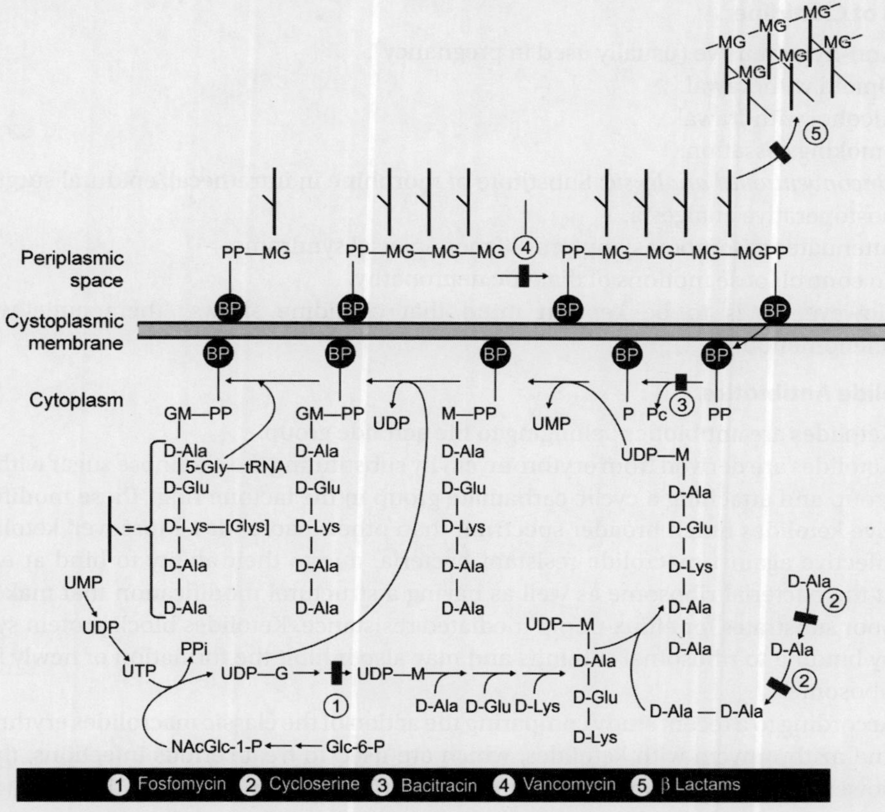

4. Smoking Cessation

The goals of pharmacotherapy are:

- To reduce craving for the reward effects of nicotine
- To suppress the physical withdrawal symptoms of nicotine

Drugs used are:

- **Nicotine transdermal patch**: Withdrawal symptoms well controlled but cravings incompletely suppressed as there is no peak
- **Nicotine chewing gum**: More useful to suppress cravings than patch
- **Varenicline**: Alpha-4-beta-2 subtype NR selective partial agonist.

  It reduces both craving by blocking reward effect pathway of nicotine as well as decreases withdrawal symptoms.
- **Bupropion**: It works by inhibiting DA and NA uptake and is rated equivalent to nicotine replacement therapy.
- **Amfebutanone**: To be used along with patch.
- **Clonidine**: Only for withdrawal.
- **Topiramate**: Glutamate receptor antagonist.
- **Glucose tablets**: Reduce craving.
- **Mecamylamine**: Nicotine antagonist.
- **Rimonabant**: Cannabinoid receptor antagonist.

5. Uses of Clonidine

- Anti-hypertensive (usually used in pregnancy).
- Opioid withdrawal.
- Alcohol withdrawal.
- Smoking cessation.
- *Unconventional analgesic*: Substitute of morphine in intrathecal/epidural surgical and postoperative analgesia.
- Attenuates vasomotor symptoms of menopausal syndrome.
- To control loose motions of diabetic neuropathy.
- However, it is to be kept in mind that clonidine shows "therapeutic window" phenomenon.

6. Ketolide Antibiotics

- Ketolides are antibiotics belonging to the acrolide group.
- Ketolides are derived from erythromycin by substituting the cladinose sugar with a keto-group and attaching a cyclic carbamate group in the lactone ring. These modifications give ketolides much broader spectrum than other macrolides. Moreover, ketolides are effective against macrolide-resistant bacteria, due to their ability to bind at two sites at the bacterial ribosome as well as having a structural modification that makes them poor substrates for efflux-pump mediated resistance. Ketolides block protein synthesis by binding to ribosomal subunits and may also inhibit the formation of newly forming ribosomes.
- According to a recent study comparing the action of the classic macrolides erythromycin and azithromycin with ketolides, which are used to treat serious infections, the more powerful drugs, i.e. ketolides were the more "leaky" in blocking the production of proteins. As a result, it is now believed that allowing cells to make some proteins could be much more damaging for a microbe than not letting it make any proteins at all. The findings may point the way to better and more potent antibiotics in future.
- The only ketolide available in the market at this moment is telithromycin. Other ketolides in development include cethromycin and solithromycin.
- *Medical use*: Community-acquired bacterial pneumonia. Other respiratory tract infections were removed as indications when it was recognized that use of telithromycin could result in hepatitis and liver failure.

7. Antidiabetic Medications according to Effect on Weight

- *Cause weight gain:*
  - Insulin
  - Sulfonylureas
- *Cause weight loss*:
  - Flozins (SGLTi)
  - GLP 1-agonists (exenatide, liraglutide)
- Weight neutral
  - Metformin
  - Gliptins (DPP4i).

8. Drugs Acting on Dopaminergic System

Subtypes	*Location*	*Function*
D1	Putamen, nucleus accumbens, i.e. nigrostrial pathway	Inhibition causes extrapyrimidal disorders
D2	Striatum, substantia nigra, pituitary	Control behavior, voluntary, prolactin release
D3	Midbrain nucleus accumbens and hypothalamus	
D4	Frontal cortex, medulla and midbrain, i.e. mesocortical pathway	
D5	Hypothalamus, hippocampus	

Significance of Dopaminergic Pathways

- *Mesolimbic pathway*: Associated with pleasure, reward and goal directed behavior
- *Mesocortical pathway*: Associated with motivational and emotional responses
- *Nigrostriatal pathway*: Involved in coordination of movement (part of basal ganglia motor loop/EPS)
- *Tuberoinfundibular pathway*: Regulates secretion of prolactin by pituitary gland and involved in maternal behavior.

Drugs Modifying Dopaminergic Transmission

Mechanism	*Drug*	*Effect*	*Use*
Synthesis	L-DOPA	↑ Synth	Parkinson disease
	2 methyl-p-tyrosine	Inhibits tyrosine hydroxylase	Expts
	Carbidopa, benserazide	Inhibit dopa decarboxylase	Parkinsonism
Storage	Reserpine, Tetrabenazine MAO inhibitors	Disrupt storage Enhance storage	Tranquilizer
Release	Amphetamine, tyramine, mazindol	Release dopamine on receptors	Anorectic, CNS stimulant
Inactivation of uptake	Amphetamine, cocaine Benztropine, benzhexol		CNS stimulant Parkinson's disease
Inactivation of metabolism	Iproniazid, tranylcypromine	Nonselective MAO inhibitors	
	Selegiline	MAO inhibitors	Parkinson's disease

Dopaminergic Pathways

- Mesolimbic pathway
- Mesocortical pathway
- Nigrostriatal pathway
- Tuberoinfundibular pathway
- Incertohypothalamic pathway

- Medullary periventricular
- Retinal.

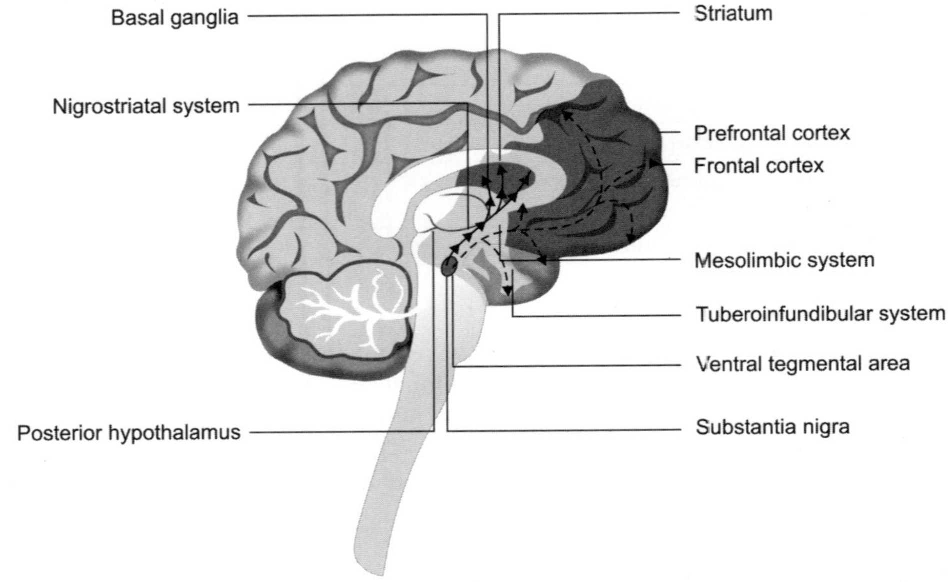

9. Drugs Acting on Serotonergic System

- **5HT precursor**: Tryptophan.
- **Synthesis inhibitor**: p-chloro-phenyl alanine.
- **Uptake inhibitor**: SSRIs (fluoxetine, etc.).
- **Storage inhibitor:** Reserpine, fenfluramine.
- **Degradation inhibitor**: Tranylcypromine, MAO inhibitor (chlorgyline).
- **Neuronal degeneration**: 5-6-dihydroxy tryptamine.

Receptor mediated

Receptor	*Agonists*	*Antagonists*
5HT 1	1A: Buspirone 1B/1D: Sumatriptan	Methysergide
5HT 2	2A/B/C: Alpha-methyl 5HT	2A: Ketanserin, cyproheptadine, risperidone 2A/C: Clozapine, methysergide
5HT 3	2-methyl 5HT	Ondansetron
5HT 4	Cisapride	Piboserod

*non selective 5HT agonist- D-lysergic acid diethylamide

10. Antitussives.

Classification

Centrally acting antitussive

- *Narcotic antitussive:*
  - Codeine

- Hydrocodone
- Oxycodone
- *Non-narcotic antitussive:*
  - Dextromethorphan
  - Noscapine
  - Propoxyphene

Peripherally acting antitussive

- *Mucosal anesthetics:*
  - Benzonatate
  - Chlophedianol
- *Hydrating agents:*
  - Steam
  - Aerosols
- *Miscellaneous:*
  - Bromhexine.

11. Disease-modifying Antirheumatic Drugs (DMARDS)

- These are slow-acting anti-rheumatic drugs
- The onset of benefit with DMARDs takes a few months of regular treatment
- Relapses occur few months after cessation of therapy.

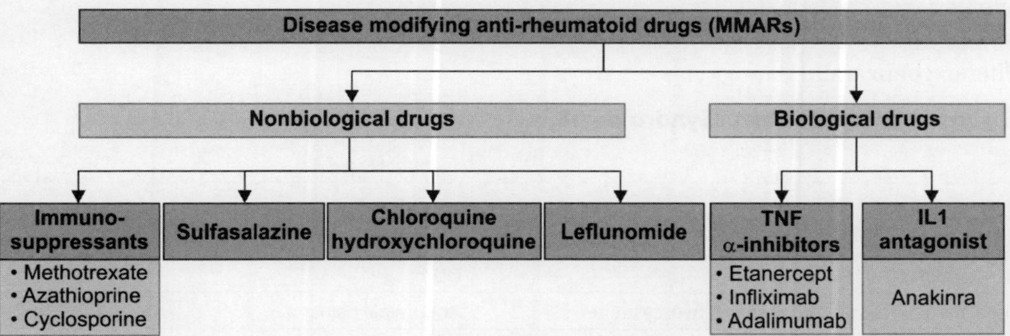

12. Drugs for Acne Vulgaris

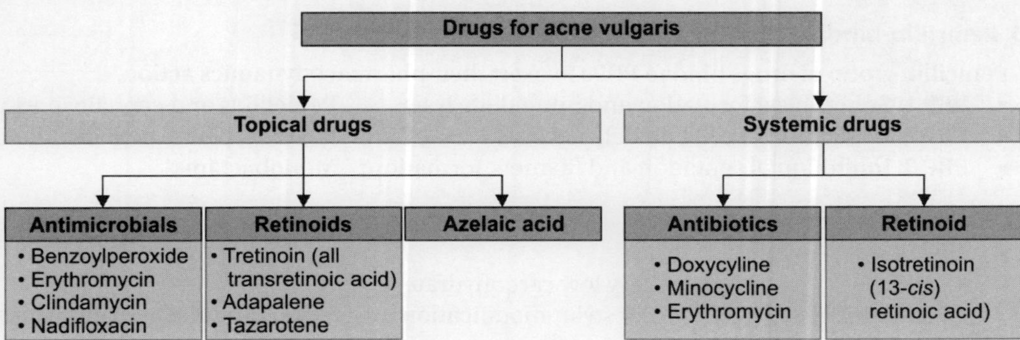

13. Drugs for Diabetes Insipidus

Nephrogenic		*Neurogenic*	
Drug	*Notes*	*Drug*	*Notes*
Amiloride	Drug of choice for Lithium induced nephrogenic DI	Vasopressin or its analogs	Drug of choice for neurogenic DI
Indomethacin	Reduces polyuria by decreasing renal PG synthesis	Carbamazepine	Unclear mechanism. Works in pituitary origin DI
		Chlorpropamide	Sensitizes kidney to ADH action

- Thiazide is the only drug that is useful both in pituitary origin as well as renal DI.

14. Drugs for Peripheral Vascular Disease

Drug	*Mechanism of action*
Cyclandelate	Papaverine like smooth muscle relaxant
Xanthinol nicotinate	Vasodilatation (combined action of xanthene and nicotinic acid)
Pentoxiphylline	Weak PDE inhibitor, reduced blood viscocity and increases RBC flexibility
Cilostazol	PDE 3 inhibitor Antiaggregatory and inodilator

Other drugs that are less commonly used:
- Isoxsuprine
- Nifedipine
- Prazosine
- Phenoxybenzamine.

15. Drugs for Irritable Bowel Syndrome (IBS)

Agent	*Symptom Relief*
Bulking agents (such as psyllium)	Constipation
Laxative	Constipation
Antispasmodics (such as loperamide)	Diarrhea
Antispasmodics (such as dicyclomine, hyoscyamine)	Abdominal pain
Antidepressants (such as tricyclic antidepressants, desipramine)	Abdominal pain
Serotonin $(5\text{-HT})_2$ receptor antagonist (such as alosetron)	Abdominal pain and diarrhea
Serotonin $(5\text{-HT})_4$ receptor partial agonist (such as tegaserod)	Constipation

16. Penicillin-binding Proteins (PBPs)

Penicillin group of drugs bind to PBPs to exert their pharmacodynamics action.
- PBP 1: Spheroblast formation and immediate lysis: Penicillins and cephalosporins
- PBP 2: Elongation of cell and delayed lysis: Reverse spectrum penicillins
- PBP 3: Inhibition of septation and filament formation: Monobactams

17. Antiobesity Therapy

- *Diet plans (A to Z):*
  - Atkins : Very low carbohydrate
  - Traditional : Lifestyle modification, exercise, attitudes, relationships, nutrition

  - Ornish : Very high carbohydrate
  - Zone : Low carbohydrate
- *Drugs:*
  - Lorcaserin
  - Phentermine + Topiramate
  - Orlistat
  - Amphetamine
  - Sibutramine
  - Rimonabant
  - Naltrexone + Bupropion
  - GLP-1 agonist (liraglutide)
- *Surgical*:
  - Bariatric surgery
  - Liposuction.

18. Current Day Uses of Thalidomide

- Multiple myeloma at initial stage
- Relapsed refractory cases of multiple myeloma
- Erythema nodosum leprosum
- Skin manifestations of systemic lupus erythematosus (SLE)
- However, for most of these indications; the congener Lenalidomide is preferred.

19. Drugs for Erectile Dysfunction

- *Orally effective drugs*:
  - *PDE V inhibition*: Sildenafil (Tadalafil is the longest acting).
  - *Apomorphine*: Dopamine agonist.
  - *Trazodone*: Antidepressant.
  - *Phentolamine*: Nonselective alpha-blocker
- *Intracavernous injection:*
  - Alprostadil
  - Thymoxamine
  - Papaverin induced penile erection (PIPE).

20. Emergency Contraception

- *Oral drugs:*
  - Levonorgestrel 0.75 mg two doses 12 hours apart or 1.5 mg single dose, taken as soon as possible; but within 72 hours of unprotected intercourse.
  - Ulipristal 30 mg single dose, as soon as possible; but within 120 hours of unprotected intercourse.
  - Mifepristone 600 mg single dose, as soon as possible; but within 72 hours of unprotected intercourse.
- Intrauterine contraceptive device (IUCD):
  - Levonorgestrel intrauterine system (LNG-IUS)
  - Cu-bearing IUCD.

Index

M

N

Q

R

S

T

W

X

Y

Z